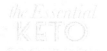

TABLE OF CONTENTS

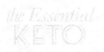

FOREWORD

Do you remember the first time you heard of the Toyota Prius?

You might have loved or hated the idea of a hybrid car. Either way, shortly after you first heard about the Prius, you probably started seeing them *everywhere*.

That's what happened to me with the ketogenic diet. And like the Prius, there's a good reason that the ketogenic diet is exploding in popularity.

When I first heard about ketosis (from The Art and Science of Low Carbohydrate Performance), I was eating a high-carb Paleo diet. And I was doing pretty well on it.

I had healed my autoimmune condition. Plus, as a professional cyclist, my performance was very good.

So I was a bit skeptical. After all, how on earth could an elite cyclist ever perform without carbohydrates?

But I just kept hearing about this diet. Every time I listened to a podcast, people were talking about this new anti-inflammatory and ultra-efficient energy source called beta-hydroxybutyrate.

And the people talking about ketosis were people I greatly respected. Tim Noakes got excited about high-fat and ketogenic diets. And then I interviewed the brilliant Dominic D'Agostino for my podcast. What he said blew me away and pushed me over the edge and into a new way of eating. We're now good friends.

I won't say that I'll never go back to eating more carbs. But I can't imagine it right now. I love having more energy than ever and especially being free from constant hunger.

My health is better than ever, and my performance on my bike is amazing. And in my practice, many of my clients also see amazing results from a ketogenic diet.

That's why I love that Louise has created this amazing cookbook. It's a tool that you can use to greatly improve your health and likely lose more than a few pounds if you want.

So what's the secret to ketosis?

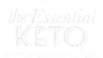

Scientists continue to look for a biochemical advantage to being in a state of ketosis, but my prediction is *there is no such advantage*.

That might sound surprising, since I'm such a huge fan of the ketogenic diet. But I believe that ketogenic diets work their magic for weight loss through *appetite suppression*.

Make no mistake, though - this appetite suppression is both a *powerful* and *dangerous* tool. It's extremely powerful if you want to lose weight. The primary reason people fail on diets is because they get hungry and can't stick to the diet.

On the other hand, appetite suppression is a bit dangerous if you are an elite athlete with no desire to lose weight. Excessive calorie restriction for extended periods of weeks or months leads to metabolic adaptations that lead to unfavorable changes in body composition. So please be wary!

Most of the people who come to me for help have very specific complaints like fatigue, insomnia, digestive and hormonal issues. For these people, I recommend putting ketosis on the backburner until we've resolved their complaints.

Often I hear back from these people months after they've finished a healing program: "I'm in ketosis, and I feel fantastic," they say. Especially the men - men always seem to do great on ketogenic diets, and by great I mean leaner, stronger and more energetic than ever.

So, if you're at the end of your healing and ready to get leaner, stronger, and regain your energy, then please let Louise's book help you – enjoy her delicious and nutritious recipes.

Remember to prioritize food quality, resist the temptation to eat high-fat dairy, avoid artificial sweeteners as much as you can, and don't forget to eat vegetables!

Luckily if you follow the recipes in this book, all of these important aspects of a ketogenic diet that most people forget about will be easy to implement as all of the recipes already take these aspects into account.

So, all that's left is for me to wish you luck and to enjoy all that extra energy you'll be living with.

Christopher Kelly
Nourish Balance Thrive
www.nourishbalancethrive.com

the Essential
KETO

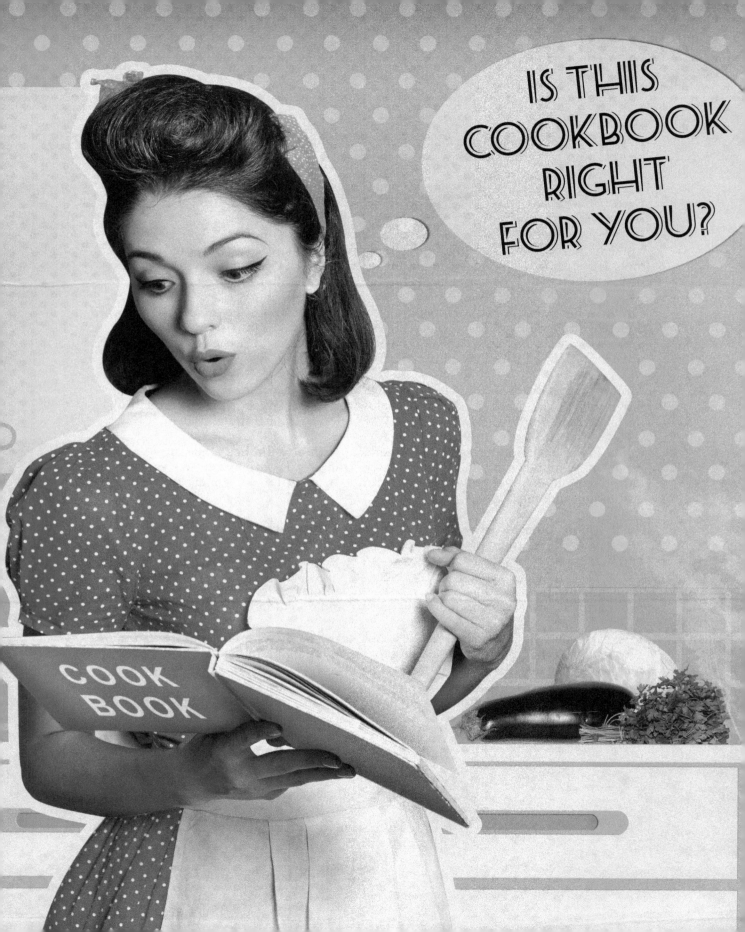

Over the past 7 years, I've helped a lot of people lose weight and heal their bodies.

I've also personally tried Low-Carb, Paleo, Gluten-Free, AIP, and Ketogenic diets.

I've always wanted to give people the best possible health information. That's why I co-founded two magazines, and the Keto Summit.

It's also why I wrote this cookbook. More readers than ever are asking me for ketogenic information and recipes.

If you're starting a ketogenic diet, you need both practical information and delicious recipes. You'll get all that and more from this cookbook.

I asked Christopher Kelly, a Certified FDN Practitioner, to write the foreword to this book. I've spent a lot of time researching ketogenic diets, but Chris is on another level.

He's a professional mountain bike racer who lives and competes on a ketogenic diet.

In this introduction, I'm going to provide you with the basics of a ketogenic diet. If you want more science behind the ketogenic diet, please check out nourishbalancethrive.com.

Now...

This cookbook is right for you if...

• You're looking for keto recipes that taste delicious and work every time.

• You want a diet that could help you lose weight without feeling like you're starving all the time.

• You want recipes that are keto AND healthy!

amounts of protein, and few carbohydrates.

But there are also many mistakes I see people make. So please make sure to read the section on page 11 titled " MISTAKES TO AVOID ON A KETOGENIC DIET."

First...

A BRIEF HISTORY OF THE KETOGENIC DIET

The ketogenic diet has gotten popular recently as an effective fat loss diet. But it was originally designed in the 1920s by Dr. Russell Wilder at the Mayo Clinic.

Dr. Wilder used ketogenic diets as an effective treatment for epilepsy in children. However, after anti-seizure medications became widely available, the ketogenic diet fell out of favor.

From 1940 until almost 1980, there was little interest in ketogenic diets.

Then, the popularity of low-carb (or Atkins) diets started to rekindle interest. And the rise of Paleo diets has prompted a full resurgence of interest in the ketogenic diet.

This time, though, the primary focus is weight loss and health.

In 2013, the ketogenic diet was the 5th most-searched-for diet on Google. Since that time, its popularity has only increased.

In fact, a clinical trial began in 2015 to test the impact of a keto diet on type 2 diabetes and pre-diabetes. The results aren't out yet, of course. Still, more research is now underway to understand the benefits of keto diets.

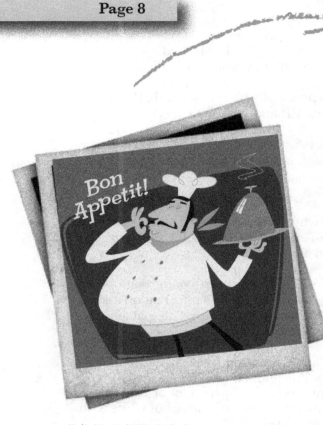

WHAT IS A KETOGENIC DIET?

A keto or ketogenic diet is a diet plan that helps your body achieve nutritional ketosis.

That means your body is relying primarily on fat and ketones (rather than sugar) for its energy. Ketones are produced when your body breaks down fat.

The cells in your body can create energy from one of four sources. They can use fat, carbohydrate, protein, or ketones.

When you go on a ketogenic diet, you force the cells in your body to primarily use fat and ketones for fuel. And there are several benefits of doing this, which I'll explain on page 10.

Most people can achieve nutritional ketosis by eating a lot of fat, moderate

Current advocates of ketogenic diets include Ben Greenfield and Jimmy Moore (author of the book, Keto Clarity).

IS A KETOGENIC DIET SAFE?

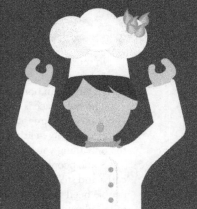

First, a quick disclaimer. I am not a doctor, medical professional, or nutritionist. Any suggestions provided in this book are not a substitute for medical or nutritional advice. You should definitely consult your physician before beginning any exercise or nutrition program.

With all that in mind, the answer is generally yes. A ketogenic diet is safe for healthy adults. But there is a lot of misinformation about keto diets. Consequently, many people will tell you that ketogenic diets are dangerous.

Here are a few quick facts you should know about the ketogenic diet and its safety:

1. Ketosis is NOT the Same as Ketoacidosis.

Many people (including medical professionals) get confused about this. Ketosis is when your body uses ketones as its primary energy source (instead of glucose).

Ketoacidosis is something altogether different. First of all, it's a serious medical condition. It usually occurs in a few different situations:

- Type 1 diabetes.
- Alcoholic binges.
- End-stage Type 2 diabetes.
- Extended periods of starvation (over the course of months).
- Prolonged severe exercise.
- A few cases of Ecstasy use have caused ketoacidosis.

In ketoacidosis, the body produces an excessive amount of ketones. That causes the blood to become acidic, which can be quite dangerous.

In a healthy adult, the body will regulate the amount of ketones produced so that this doesn't happen. For instance, the body will release insulin to stop the burning of fats.

Eating a ketogenic diet or even fasting for a few days will NOT cause an overload of ketones.

2. Carbohydrates are NOT Essential for the Human Body.

This is another common misconception.

Protein, some fats, and many vitamins and minerals are essential for the human body. Carbohydrates, however, are not essential.

Cells that lack a mitochondrion (such as some very small neurons and red blood cells) always need a small amount of glucose. But even in ketosis, your body can easily fill those needs by turning protein into glucose.

This is how you can live for 40-60 days without eating. Your body converts fat stores into ketones, which your body then uses for energy.

3. Pay Attention to Your Gut Health

Over the years, this is one of the biggest mistakes I've seen people make.

Meat and seafood are great, but your gut won't thrive on those foods alone. You must make sure to eat plenty of vegetables that are high in fiber to support your gut.

The bacteria and other microorganisms in your gut need fiber and resistant starch to do their job.

So besides fibrous veggies, also consume probiotics and fermented foods on a regular basis.

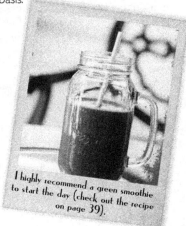

I highly recommend a green smoothie to start the day (check out the recipe on page 39).

KETO VS LOW CARB

In most ways, a ketogenic diet is very similar to a low carb diet. In particular, you must restrict carbohydrates in both diets.

The difference is that a ketogenic diet is all about making sure that your body is in ketosis. While eating low-carb is a big part of that, it's not the only thing you should think about.

Some people can eat a high amount of daily carbs and still be in nutritional ketosis. Other people need to eat many fewer carbs and also make other adjustments to achieve the same state. Men usually seem to have it easier than women in this respect.

I like to think of a ketogenic diet as a more precise version of a low carb diet. You're paying closer attention to what's going on in your body. Rather than focusing only on how many carbs you eat, you're ensuring that your body is burning fat for energy.

But please don't get stuck on the labels. In the end, you can be on a low carb, ketogenic, or even Paleo diet, and still be eating exactly the same foods!

Each diet places a slight emphasis on a different aspect of what you eat, but the results can be identical.

Most people would consider every recipe in this cookbook to be Ketogenic, Low Carb, and Paleo (as well as dairy-free, grain-free, and gluten-free!).

My best suggestion is to forget about the classifications. Instead, ask yourself these questions about the food you eat:

What is this food doing for or to my body?

Does this food provide me with nutrients (e.g., vitamins, minerals, essential amino acids, etc.)?

Does this food contain toxins (gluten, processed sugar, etc.) that could prevent my body from functioning well?

Does this food hinder my body from staying in ketosis?

WILL A KETOGENIC DIET HELP ME LOSE WEIGHT?

A ketogenic diet is not magic. Without a doubt, some people have more success than others. So I can't guarantee any particular results.

However, I have seen many people lose a lot of weight with ketogenic diets. And I truly believe that a ketogenic diet is one of the most effective and healthiest ways to lose weight.

There are a few big reasons why ketogenic diets work so well...

1. Controlling Hunger

This is the single biggest reason that ketogenic diets are great. And it's also the biggest reason that most other diets fail.

Ketogenic diets help your body's regulation of hormones and neurotransmitters. One of the results is that you get much less hungry.

That means reduced cravings for junk food, less cheating, and more weight loss.

If you've ever dieted before, then you know that sticking to it is the hardest part. Sticking to a ketogenic diet is much easier, because you don't face the same hunger.

2. Metabolic Flexibility

If you've been eating a high-carb diet, then your body is excellent at burning carbohydrates for energy.

That makes sense when you're eating a lot of carbs. But it also means that your body is often not good at burning fat.

Ideally, your body should be able to switch back and forth between burning carbs and fat. When your body can't do this, it's called "poor metabolic flexibility."

In that case, you don't burn much fat, you get cravings for sugar and carbs, and you have a hard time losing weight. That's one of the reasons that you might get hungrier on a high-carb diet. If your body can't burn fat well, then you'll be hungry whenever your blood sugar is low.

A ketogenic diet can help you regain metabolic flexibility. By putting your body into a state of ketosis, you force your body to get better at burning fat.

And many people find that they end up burning a lot of their bodies' fat stores, which is exactly what you want for weight loss.

3. Hyper-Palatability

You might have never heard of hyper-palatable foods. Yet nothing has contributed to obesity more in modern times.

A food is hyper-palatable when it has a "magic" combination of fat, sugar, and salt. The result is that foods become addictive. You can't stop eating them, even if you're full.

And food manufacturers make use of that combination to create irresistible processed foods. From potato chips to cookies to donuts, humans have created a thousand addictive foods.

But none of these foods occur in nature. Fruits usually have sugar, and meats usually have fat, but you don't find foods with both.

By removing refined carbohydrates, a ketogenic diet also removes hyper-palatable foods. And that means you won't feel an unstoppable need to keep eating and eating.

The result is that most people feel less hungry and have fewer cravings.

This means you're effortlessly restricting your calorie intake, leading to more weight loss.

4. Inflammation and Toxins

Finally, a ketogenic diet also helps you to remove toxins and reduce inflammation.

You may not even see or be aware of chronic inflammation. But inflammation in your body is a big obstacle to weight loss.

And the main causes of inflammation are many of the foods you eat. The biggest culprits are wheat and other grains, milk, and processed sugar.

Coincidentally, these are all foods that you must avoid on a ketogenic diet.

MISTAKES TO AVOID ON A KETOGENIC DIET

In this section, I want to cover some of the mistakes that I often see people make on a ketogenic diet. If you can avoid these mistakes, then you'll be much more likely to lose weight and feel better.

Mistake #1: Bad Mindset

Many people treat the ketogenic diet as something they'll "try for a week or two."

They want to dip their toe in the water to see if the diet "works." But they definitely don't want to commit.

There are two problems with this approach. First of all, if you're not committed, then you're going to give up at the first sign of trouble. If you get tempted, or if you don't lose weight for a few days, then you'll give it all up. And I can guarantee that not everything will go perfectly for you. It never does.

The second problem is that no diet works unless you approach it as a lifestyle.

If you want, you can lose some weight and then go back to eating bread, pasta, and sugar. But if you go back to eating those foods, you'll also go back to gaining weight. That is what we call the yo-yo dieting trap.

Mistake #2: Eating Too Much Protein

By all means, you need to eat enough protein. It's also easy, though, to eat too much protein.

Keeping your carbs low is the most important way to cause ketosis. Unfortunately, eating too much protein can also prevent your body from going into ketosis.

Mistake #3: Not Testing

Our bodies are all a little bit different. Two people eating the same ketogenic diet can sometimes get different results.

One person could be in ketosis and losing weight, and another person could be struggling.

That's why testing is so important. You need to make sure that you're actually in ketosis. And if you aren't, then you can make adjustments to your diet and life.

When you're in ketosis, your body will produce ketone bodies. There are 3 types of ketone bodies: Acetoacetate (AcAc), Beta-hydroxybutyrate (BHB), and Acetone.

In your blood, you can measure all 3 ketone bodies. In

your urine, AcAc and Acetone can be measured. And in your breath, just Acetone.

Your blood ketone levels are the best indicator of ketosis. Unfortunately, measuring blood ketone levels is also the most expensive method.

That's why many people still measure their urine and breath ketone levels instead.

No matter which method you use, test more frequently in the beginning. Once you're in ketosis, you won't need to test as often, because your body will more easily stay in ketosis.

Another great test to consider is a DEXA scan. This test will measure your fat levels as well as your bone and muscle levels. If you do it before you start your diet, you'll be able to later track precisely how well your diet is working.

Mistake #4: Not Eating Enough Nutrient-Dense Foods

On a ketogenic diet, you'll pay a lot of attention to the macronutrients you eat. Getting the right proportion of fats, carbs, and protein is very important.

But don't forget that you also need to be getting enough vitamins and minerals.

You might be aware of some terrible things that happen if you're severely deficient in a micronutrient. For example...

• You can get scurvy if you don't get enough vitamin C.

• You can get goiter if you're deficient in iodine.

• Or you could go blind if you don't get enough vitamin A.

Besides those acute problems, chronic deficiencies can also be a huge problem. Often, nutrient deficiencies are not so severe that you exhibit a particular disease. That doesn't mean, though, that they're not making you less healthy.

Over time, if you're low in vitamins and minerals, your body just won't function well. That can lead to illnesses, fatigue, and more. Even minor vitamin and mineral deficiencies might be making it harder for you to lose weight.

An easy way to boost your micronutrient

intake is to eat more nutrient-dense foods. Most of these foods fit well into a ketogenic diet.

For instance, green leafy vegetables, organ meats, and seafood are all ketogenic-friendly. And they're some of the most nutrient-dense foods you can eat.

Supplementation with a good multivitamin is also helpful.

If you're into testing, then try getting a SpectraCell analysis or an Urine Organic Acid test. Both of these tests will tell you which vitamins and minerals you're deficient in. That way, you can focus specifically on those deficiencies.

Mistake #5: Eating Toxic, Inflammatory Foods - Even if They're Low Carb

Not everything that is low in carbs is good for you. Period.

For example, you can go to most grocery stores these days and find low-carb processed foods. You can get low-carb bread, low-carb cookies, and low-carb snacks.

You might be able to stay in ketosis while eating those low-carb foods, but they're still bad for your body. Many of them contain wheat, gluten, and other inflammatory ingredients.

And as I mentioned, inflammation always makes it harder for you to lose weight.

Here are ingredients that I suggest avoiding, even in low-carb foods:

• Wheat, Rye, and Barley. New technology has created a way to make these foods low-carb sometimes. But they still always contain gluten, which will inevitably cause inflammation in your body. Plus, they're not very nutrient-dense.

• Dairy. Yes - even cheese. In the abstract, dairy might be ok. The problem is that you don't live in an abstract world. Milk will pretty much always keep you out of ketosis. And the vast majority of people have some level of sensitivity to dairy products like cheese. (This is most likely true even if you aren't lactose-intolerant.)

• Vegetable and Seed Oils. This includes Vegetable Oil, Canola Oil, Corn Oil, Sunflower Oil, and similar products. Your cooking oil also makes a huge difference to your weight loss. As Dr. Shanahan points out in her book, Deep Nutrition, the production of these oils produces trans-fats, which can block your enzymes for burning fat.

• Any food you have an intolerance to. Start paying more attention to your body. If you wake up one day and notice that you're congested or that your joints are stiff, ask yourself what you ate. You're likely sensitive to one of the foods you ate the day before.

Also, be careful with nuts. Many people have allergies or sensitivities to nuts. But more than that, nuts are easy to overeat. Again, a ketogenic diet is not magic, so eating 3,000 calories of nuts per day is going to make a difference.

Mistake #6: Ignoring Sleep, Exercise, and Stress

While eating a good diet is important for weight loss, it's not all that matters.

Many weight-loss studies have stressed the importance of sleep (7+ hours), exercise, and de-stressing. It's tough to get everything right all at once. Still, any small efforts you make in these areas will pay off in the end.

Mistake #7: Not Being Patient

It can take up to two or three weeks to become keto-adapted. So if you're going to give the ketogenic diet a try, then actually give it a try and be patient.

It's taken you a lifetime of eating poorly to get to where you're at. You can't expect to fix all that damage in just a few weeks.

Mistake #8: Not Eating Enough Fiber

Mainstream nutrition has gotten a lot of things wrong.

The importance of fiber is not one of them. The past few years of scientific research has shown just how important fiber is for your gut health.

In particular, soluble fiber and resistant starches from vegetables can improve your gut bacteria. Fermented foods like sauerkraut are also excellent in this regard.

WHAT IF A KETOGENIC DIET DOESN'T HELP ME LOSE WEIGHT?

This is a fear that I hear all the time...

"What if I put in all this effort - give up all these foods - and it still doesn't work?"

I completely understand this fear. I used to ask myself the same thing.

But this is also the reason why I don't believe in "dieting." Dieting is a short term project where your only goal is to lose weight.

I'm not saying that you shouldn't try to lose weight. I think it's often a worthwhile goal.

But if that's your only goal, then you'll be disappointed if you go even a few days without any results. And in the world of weight loss, you will definitely have times when you stall a little bit.

A more practical way of thinking is to focus on doing the right things, rather than just on the results. Make it your goal every day to feed your body foods that give it energy, vitamins, and minerals.

Appreciate every healthy food you eat, knowing that it will give you lasting health. In that way, you'll naturally lose weight, keep it off, and gain better health as a result.

That's why this cookbook isn't just about replacing the carbs in your diet with other junk.

This is not just another low carb cookbook.

Instead, this cookbook will help you focus on the principles behind the ketogenic diet. (And, of course, provide you with delicious ketogenic foods as well.)

I want you to lose weight. But I also want you to enjoy nutrient-dense and delicious foods that are low in toxins.

That way, there's no downside to eating recipes from this cookbook. Even if you don't lose weight immediately, you're still feeding your body nourishing foods.

At this point you might be thinking, "yeah, but what do I do if I still don't lose weight?"

I've helped thousands of people - through our website, magazines, and otherwise. So I won't lie to you and say that it never happens. Sometimes, someone will have an abnormally hard time losing weight.

If you're doing everything right but aren't getting results, then something else is going on in your body that you are not aware of. That's when I recommend you do some extensive testing with someone like Christopher Kelly.

It could be something as simple as having a gut pathogen. Or it could be something more complex like hypothyroidism or autoimmune disorders.

The point is this.

Diet is perhaps the most important part of losing weight. But it's still only a part. If your body is using energy and resources on an underlying health condition, weight loss is much harder.

However, in 98% of cases, getting your diet and lifestyle in order is enough. So don't jump to the conclusion that you have other issues.

WHAT CAN I EAT ON A KETOGENIC DIET?

Eat plenty of fats, moderate amounts of protein, and very little carbohydrates.

Carbohydrate Intake:

In Keto Clarity, Jimmy Moore suggests eating less than 100g per day of carbohydrates. For most people, that number needs to be under 50g. For people with insulin resistance, you might need to consume under 30g or 20g per day.

If you are a serious athlete, then your carbohydrate intake may need to be higher than even 100g per day.

Estimated nutritional information is provided for every recipe in this cookbook to help you plan your meals. Our meal plan has been designed to provide 20g or less of net carbohydrates per day per person.

To make it easier for you to get an estimate as to how much you should be eating, try using our Keto Calculator here: http://paleomagazine.com/keto-calculator

Please note that this calculator is designed only as a guide to how much you should be eating.

WHAT'S DIFFERENT ABOUT THIS COOKBOOK?

This cookbook contains recipes that will help you get into nutritional ketosis.

But as I pointed out above, a variety of other factors will determine if you're actually in ketosis. So, no matter what you eat, you might need to do some tweaking.

Nonetheless, these recipes (which are grain-free, soy-free, dairy-free, peanut-free, and free of seed oils) will help you reach ketosis while also providing your body with nutrient-dense meals to satisfy your hunger and heal your body.

Quick Note about Tamari Sauce, Ghee, Sesame Oil, and Stevia:

These are 4 ingredients that people often ask about. This book doesn't go into the science and ideas behind the keto diet, but you can read about why these 4 ingredients are ok to use on a keto diet here (and if you're not familiar with those ingredients, then those articles also explain what they are):

Tamari Sauce article -
http://paleomagazine.com/is-tamari-sauce-paleo
Ghee article -
http://paleomagazine.com/is-ghee-paleo
Sesame Oil article -
http://paleomagazine.com/is-sesame-oil-paleo
Stevia article -
http://paleomagazine.com/what-is-stevia-and-should-you-eat-it

If for any reason you'd prefer not to use these 4 ingredients, you can:

- use Coconut Aminos instead of Tamari Sauce
- use Coconut Oil instead of Ghee
- use Olive Oil instead of Sesame Oil, and
- omit Stevia from the recipe.

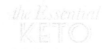

FOUR TIPS FOR MEAL PLANNING ON A KETOGENIC DIET

There's a 2-week meal plan at the back of this book along with a ketogenic diet food list. That meal plan is designed to provide 20g or less of net carbs per day. If you received our additional 4-week Keto meal plan, then that plan also uses recipes from this cookbook.

But I know everybody's tastes and lifestyles are different, so if you want to do your own meal planning, then here are four tips to help make your life easier:

1. Keep it simple

It's easy to fall off a diet if preparing the meals gets too complicated. So, remember to keep it simple. I love cooking a large batch of meat in the slow cooker, such as the slow cooker chicken and bacon or the oxtail stew. Then, we eat it over the next few days - each time with some veggie side dishes.

Or, for more variation, we sauté the meat with whatever veggies we have on hand. Or, we throw it into some bone broth with some veggies and make a quick soup out of it.

2. Eat the same foods on multiple days

It's easy to use up all your mental energy trying to figure out what to eat. Another way to keep it simple is to eat the same foods on multiple days. Breakfast is an easy meal to do this with. During the weekdays, choose an easy and nutritious breakfast recipe to make every day. The coconut ghee coffee (page 194) or the breakfast green smoothie (page 39) are both excellent options to start your day with.

3. Plan what you'll eat if you get stuck at work or can't eat at home

Many diets fail because you had one bad day at work, you went out to a restaurant with friends, or you went on vacation. At those times, all your great intentions vanish into thin air.

So try to plan ahead for those situations. Which local restaurant can you go to and order a steak and salad if you get home too late or you're too tired to cook?

Or if you're going out with friends, do you know exactly what you can order at the restaurant? That way, you don't even have to look at the menu again and get tempted.

4. Carry some snacks round with you

I suggest snacks like nuts, coconut butter, cacao nibs, or 100% dark chocolate to keep with you. If you do get hungry, then you can eat some of your snack rather than be tempted by foods that will derail your ketogenic diet. Just note that nuts, coconut butter, cacao nibs, and dark chocolate all do contain small amounts of net carbohydrates, so try not to overeat them!

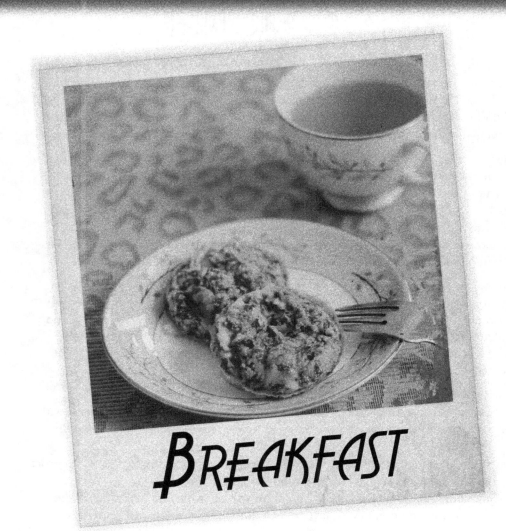

BREAKFAST

CHAPTER I

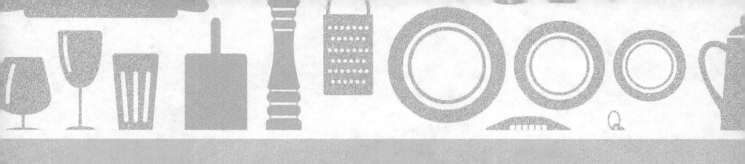

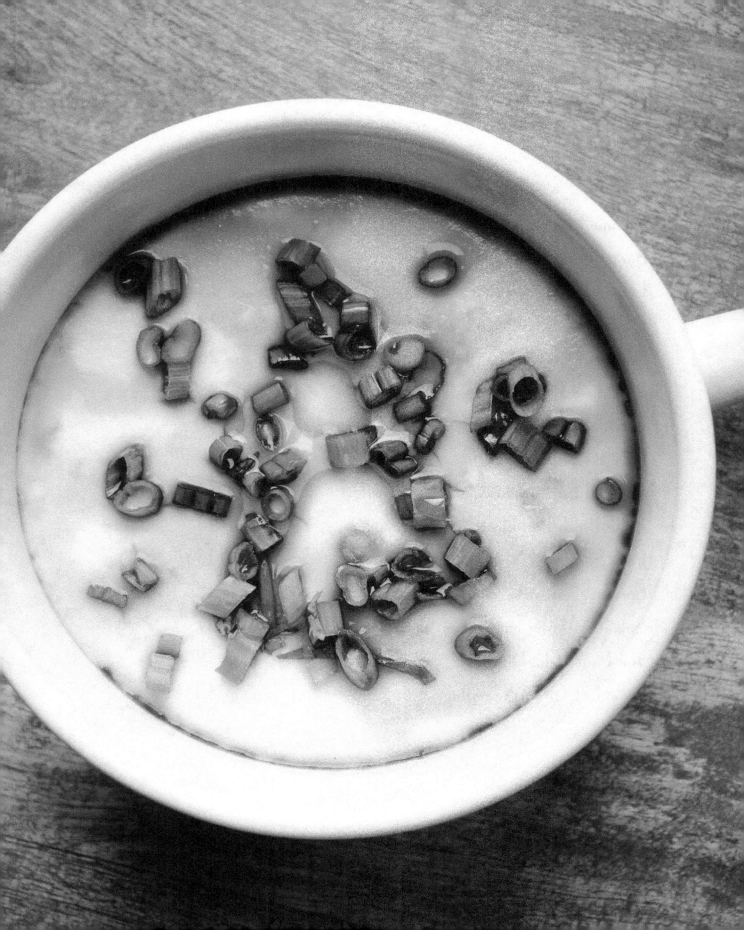

STEAMED EGG CUSTARD

Prep Time: 5 minutes
Cook Time: 15 minutes
Total Time: 20 minutes
Yield: 1 serving
Serving Size: 1 bowl

INGREDIENTS

- 2 eggs
- Room-temperature water
- 1 Tablespoon *(15 ml)* tamari sauce
- 1 teaspoon *(5 ml)* sesame oil
- 1 Tablespoon *(4 g)* scallions (chopped green onions)

This is a traditional Chinese dish that I have always loved. If you're worried about using sesame oil or tamari sauce, then please read my note on page 14. If you want to skip those ingredients, then add in some hot sauce and salt instead.

INSTRUCTIONS

1. Place the 2 eggs into a small bowl. Add room-temperature water (approx. same volume as the eggs).
2. Mix well.
3. Remove the foam that forms at the top of the bowl.
4. Place into a steamer (the water in the steamer should be boiling already) for 10-12 minutes.
5. Check to make sure the middle of the custard isn't a liquid anymore. Cook for a few minutes longer if necessary.
6. Serve with tamari sauce, sesame oil, and scallions as toppings.

SUGGESTIONS

If you don't have a steamer, don't worry, you can make your own steamer by using a tall saucepan and an old bowl. Fill the saucepan 1/3 of the way with water, place the old bowl upside down in the saucepan so that it's almost submerged in the water, and then place the bowl or plate you want to steam on top of the old bowl. Make sure the lid to the saucepan still fits and you're ready to go.

Nutritional Data (estimates) - per serving:
Calories: 170   Fat: 13 g   Net Carbohydrates: 2 g   Protein: 13 g

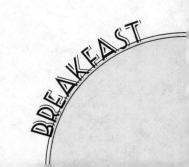

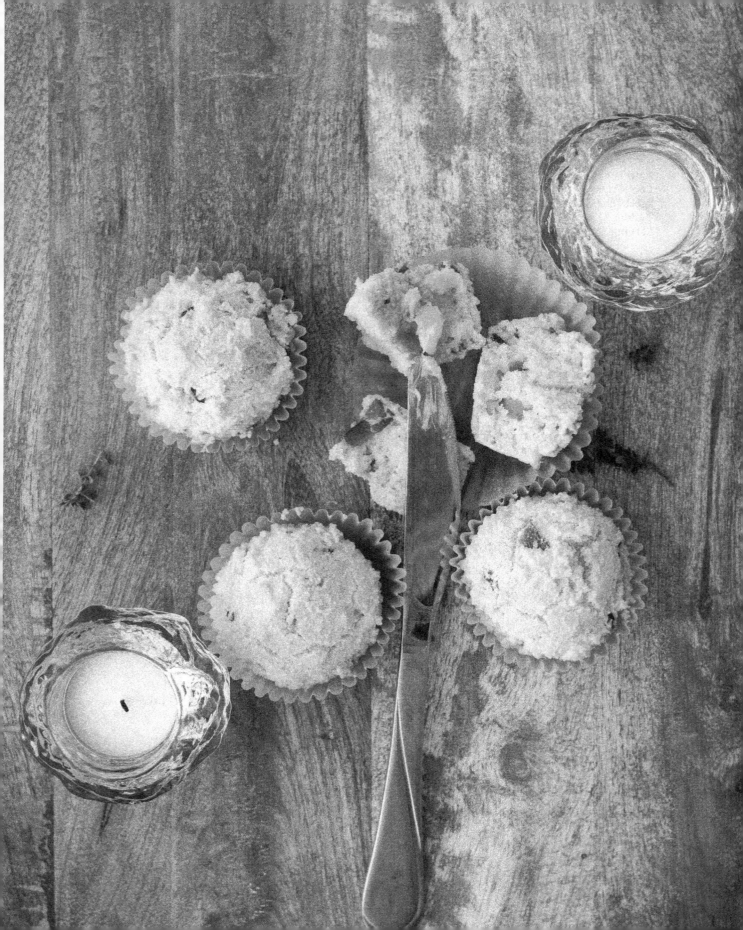

BACON LEMON THYME MUFFINS

Prep Time: 10 minutes
Cook Time: 20 minutes
Total Time: 30 minutes
Yield: 12 muffins
Serving Size: 1 muffin

While these muffins are delicious, I would advise you to not go overboard with nut flour baked goods - they're easy to overeat and high in polyunsaturated fats that can be damaged when cooked and lead to oxidative damage in our bodies.

INGREDIENTS

- 3 cups *(360 g)* almond flour
- 1 cup *(100 g)* bacon bits
- 1/2 cup *(120 ml)* ghee (or coconut oil), melted
- 4 eggs, whisked
- 2 teaspoons *(2 g)* lemon thyme (or use another herb of your choice)
- 1 teaspoon *(4 g)* baking soda
- 1/2 teaspoon *(2 g)* salt (optional)

INSTRUCTIONS

1. Preheat oven to 350 F *(175 C)*.
2. Melt the ghee in a mixing bowl.
3. Add in the rest of the ingredients except the bacon bits to the mixing bowl.
4. Mix everything together well.
5. Lastly, add in the bacon bits.
6. Line a muffin pan with muffin liners. Spoon the mixture into the muffin pan (to around 3/4 full).
7. Bake for 18-20 minutes until a toothpick comes out clean when you insert it into a muffin.

Nutritional Data (estimates) - per serving:
Calories: 300   Fat: 28 g   Net Carbohydrates: 4 g   Protein: 11 g

the Essential
KETO

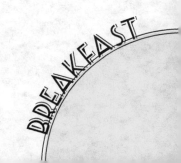

BREAKFAST

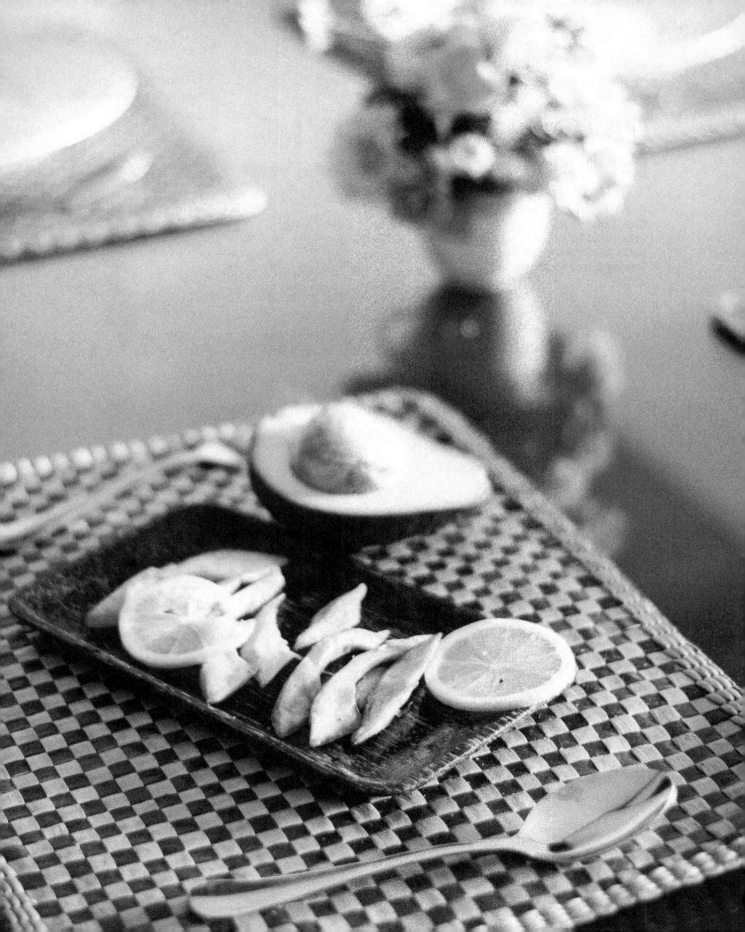

LEMON FRIED AVOCADOS

Prep Time: 2 minutes
Cook Time: 5 minutes
Total Time: 7 minutes
Yield: 2 servings
Serving Size: 1 small plate

Make sure to keep an eye on these as they burn quickly!

INGREDIENTS

- 1 ripe avocado (not too soft), cut into slices
- 1 Tablespoon *(15 ml)* coconut oil
- 1 Tablespoon *(15 ml)* lemon juice
- Salt to taste (or lemon salt)

INSTRUCTIONS

1. Add the coconut oil to a frying pan. Place the avocado slices into the oil gently.
2. Fry the avocado slices (turning them gently) so that all sides are slightly browned.
3. Sprinkle the lemon juice and salt over the slices and serve warm.

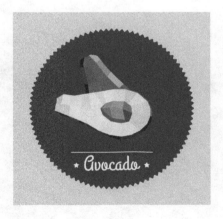

Avocado

Nutritional Data (estimates) - per serving:
Calories: 200   Fat: 20 g   Net Carbohydrates: 2 g   Protein: 2 g

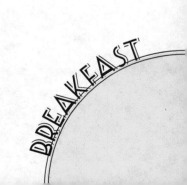

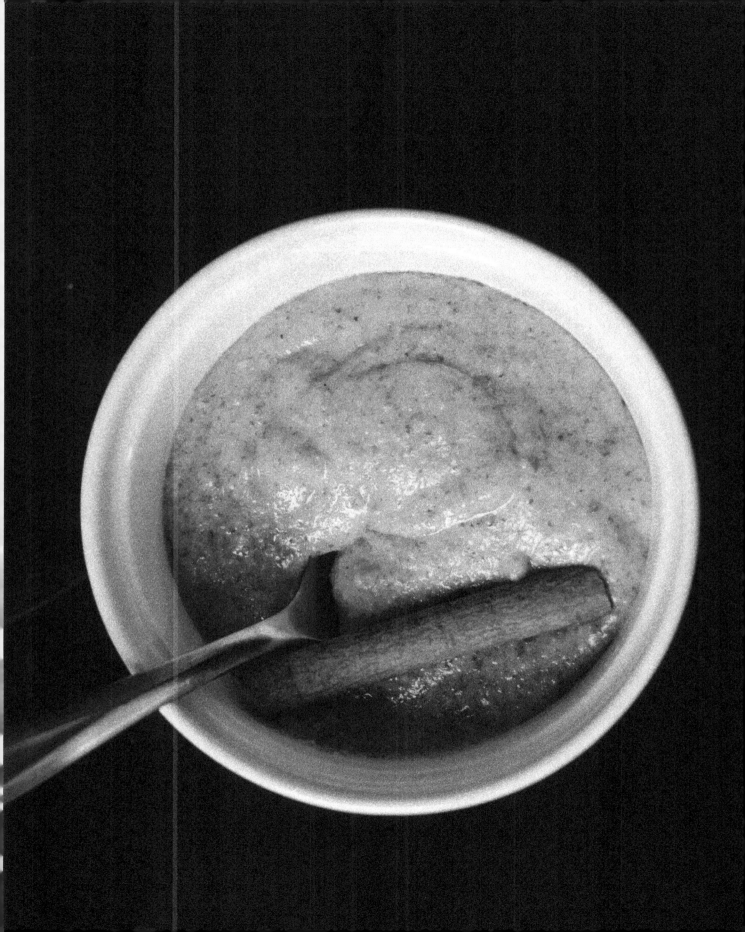

CREAMY BREAKFAST PORRIDGE

Prep Time: 2 minutes
Cook Time: 5 minutes
Total Time: 7 minutes
Yield: 2 servings
Serving Size: 1 cup

INGREDIENTS

- 1/2 cup *(60 g)* almonds, ground using a food processor or blender
- 3/4 cup *(180 ml)* coconut milk
- Stevia to taste (optional)
- 1 teaspoon *(2 g)* cinnamon powder
- Dash of nutmeg
- Dash of cloves
- Dash of cardamom (optional)

INSTRUCTIONS

1. Heat the coconut milk in a small saucepan on medium heat until it forms a liquid.
2. Add in the ground almonds and sweetener and stir to mix in.
3. Keep stirring for approximately 5 minutes (it'll start to thicken a bit more).
4. Add in the spices (have a taste to check whether you want more sweetener or spices) and serve hot.

Nutritional Data (estimates) - per serving:
Calories: 430   Fat: 40 g   Net Carbohydrates: 6 g   Protein: 8 g

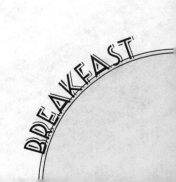

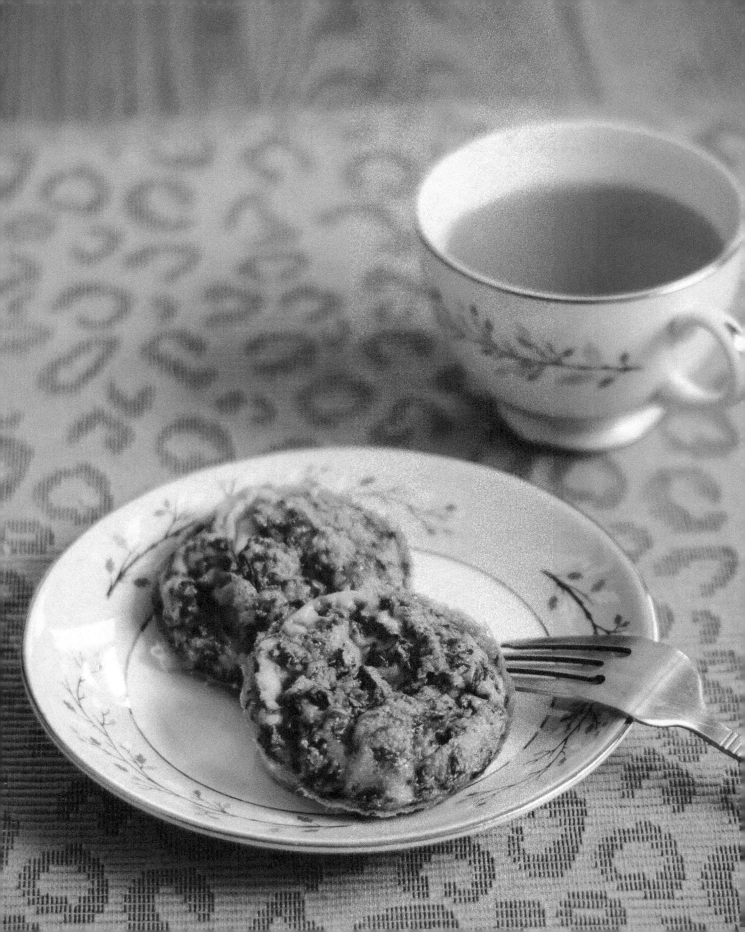

KALE AND CHIVES EGG MUFFINS

Prep Time: 10 minutes
Cook Time: 30 minutes
Total Time: 40 minutes
Yield: 4 servings
Serving Size: 2 muffins

INGREDIENTS

- 6 eggs
- 1 cup kale, finely chopped
- 1/4 cup *(17 g)* chives, finely chopped
- 1/2 cup *(120 ml)* almond or coconut milk
- Salt and pepper to taste
- 8 slices of prosciutto or bacon (optional)

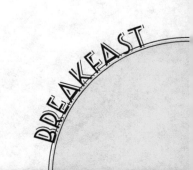

INSTRUCTIONS

1. Preheat the oven to 350 F *(175 C)*.
2. Whisk the eggs and add in the chopped kale and chives. Also add in the almond/coconut milk, salt, and pepper. Mix well.
3. Grease 8 muffin cups with coconut oil or line each cup with a prosciutto slice.
4. Divide the egg mixture between the 8 muffin cups. Fill only ⅔ of each cup as the mixture rises when it's baking.
5. Bake in oven for 30 minutes.
6. Let cool a few minutes and then lift out carefully with a fork. Note that the muffins will sink a bit.

Nutritional Data (estimates) - per serving:
Calories: 240   Fat: 20 g   Net Carbohydrates: 3 g   Protein: 12 g

BREAKFAST

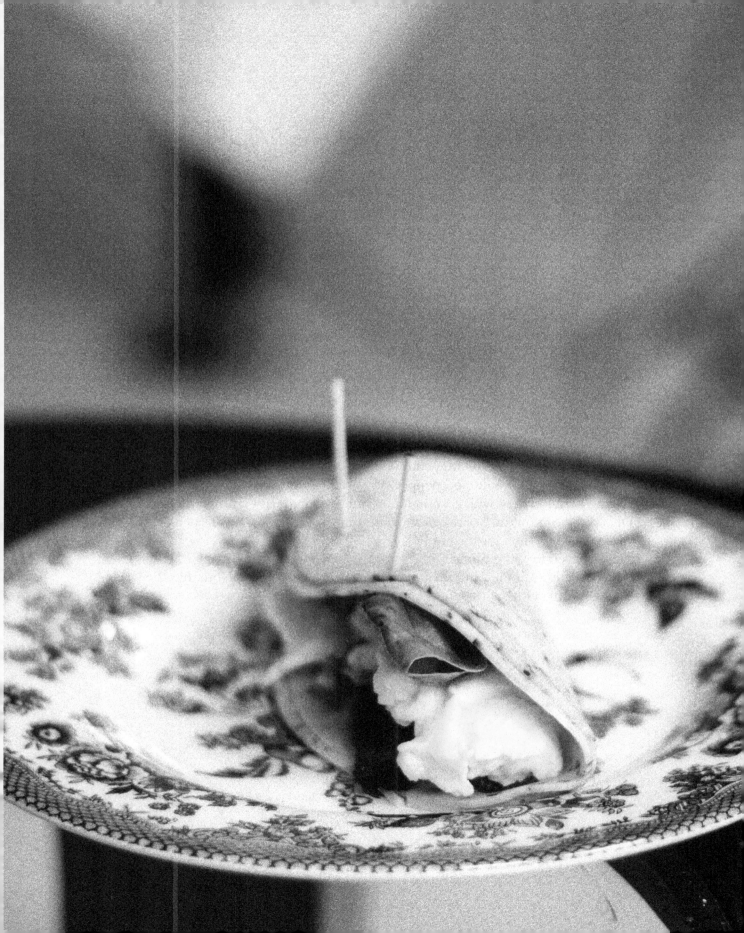

BREAKFAST TURKEY WRAP

Prep Time: 5 minutes
Cook Time: 20 minutes
Total Time: 25 minutes
Yield: 1 serving
Serving Size: 2 wraps

Wraps are hard to come by on the ketogenic diet, so be creative and try using sliced deli meat as a wrap for various foods.

INGREDIENTS

- 2 slices of turkey breast (use more if the slices break easily)
- 2 romaine lettuce leaves (or 2 slices of avocado)
- 2 slices of bacon
- 2 eggs
- 1 Tablespoon *(15 ml)* coconut oil to cook in

INSTRUCTIONS

1. Cook the 2 slices of bacon to the crispness you like.
2. Scramble the 2 eggs in the coconut oil (or bacon fat).
3. Make 2 wraps by placing half the scrambled eggs, 1 slice of bacon, and 1 romaine lettuce leaf on each slice of turkey breast.

Nutritional Data (estimates) - per serving:
Calories: 360   Fat: 30 g   Net Carbohydrates: 3 g   Protein: 20 g

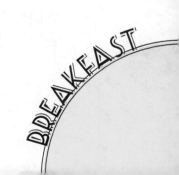

GUACAMOLE TOPPED SCRAMBLED EGGS

Prep Time: 5 minutes
Cook Time: 5 minutes
Total Time: 10 minutes
Yield: 1 serving
Serving Size: 1 bowl

INGREDIENTS

- 3 eggs
- 1 Tablespoon *(15 ml)* coconut oil
- 1/4 cup *(55 g)* guacamole (see page 187 for recipe)
- Salt to taste

INSTRUCTIONS

1. Place the coconut oil into a pan. Add the eggs and scramble over a low heat.
2. Place the scrambled eggs into a bowl and top with the guacamole. Add salt to taste.

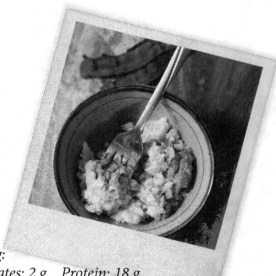

Nutritional Data (estimates) - per serving:
Calories: 370   Fat: 23 g   Net Carbohydrates: 2 g   Protein: 18 g

EASY BACON CUPS

Prep Time: 15 minutes
Cook Time: 25 minutes
Total Time: 40 minutes
Yield: 4 servings
Serving Size: 2 bacon cups

Fill these bacon cups up with some guacamole, a poached egg, scrambled eggs, or the Spinach, Mushroom, Bacon Saute (see page 37 for recipe).

INGREDIENTS
- 20 thin slices of bacon
- Equipment: standard nonstick metal muffin or cupcake pan

INSTRUCTIONS
1. Preheat oven to 400 F *(200 C)*.
2. Each bacon cup will require 2 and 1/2 slices of bacon, to be used as described in Step #3 below.
3. Start by turning the entire muffin/cupcake pan over, so that the side that is normally the bottom is on top. To make 1 bacon cup, place 2 half slices of bacon across the back of one of the muffin/cupcake cups, both in the same direction. Then, place another half slice across those 2, perpendicular to the direction of the first 2 half slices. Finally, wrap a whole slice of bacon tightly around the sides of the cup. The slice wrapped around the sides will help to hold the bottom pieces of bacon together.
4. Repeat Step #3 for the other cups. *(You can scale this recipe to as many cups as your pan has by simply using more bacon.)*
5. Place the entire pan *(still upside-down)* into the oven and bake for 25 minutes until crispy *(place a baking tray underneath in the oven to catch any dripping bacon fat)*.
6. Cool for 5-10 minutes, and then carefully remove the bacon cups from the muffin tray.

Nutritional Data (estimates) - per serving:
Calories: 180   Fat: 18 g   Net Carbohydrates: 0 g   Protein: 5 g

BREAKFAST

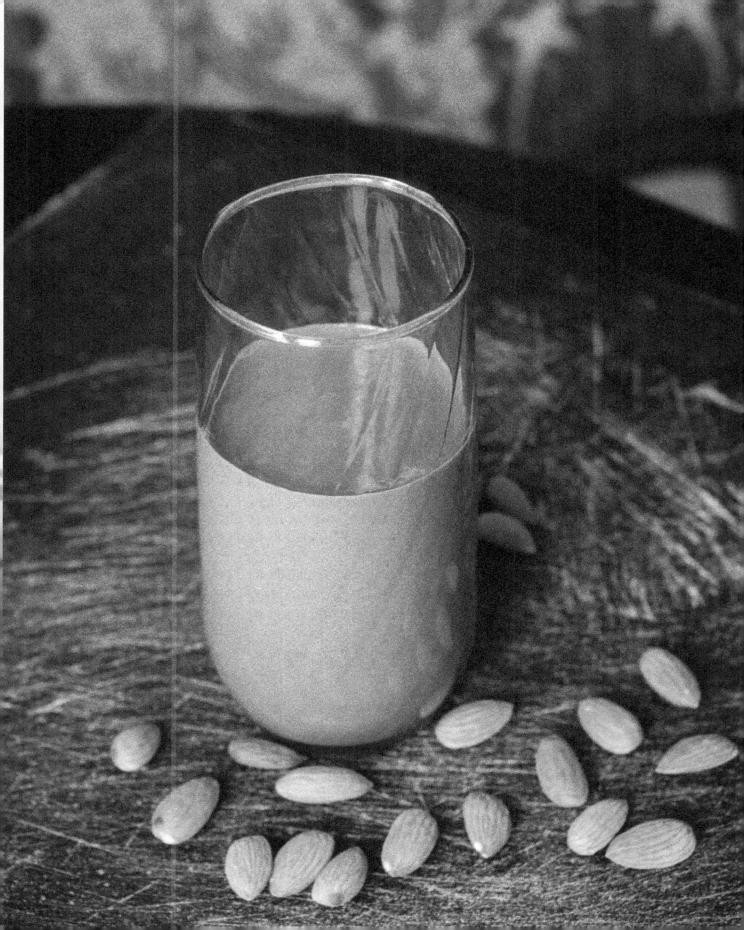

ALMOND BUTTER CHOCOLATE SHAKE

Prep Time: 5 minutes
Cook Time: 0 minutes
Total Time: 5 minutes
Yield: 1 serving
Serving Size: 1 cup

INGREDIENTS

- 1 cup *(240 ml)* coconut milk or almond milk (from cartons or dilute the canned coconut milk)
- 2 Tablespoons *(10 g)* unsweetened cacao powder
- 1 Tablespoon *(16 g)* almond butter
- 1 teaspoon *(5 ml)* vanilla extract
- 1/4 cup *(35 g)* ice (optional)
- Stevia to taste (optional)

INSTRUCTIONS

1. Place all the ingredients into a blender and blend well.

Nutritional Data (estimates) - per serving:
Calories: 190   Fat: 15 g   Net Carbohydrates: 7 g   Protein: 4 g

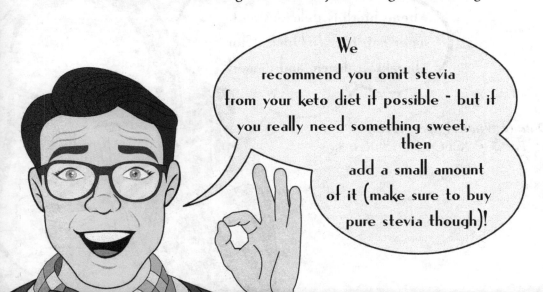

We recommend you omit stevia from your keto diet if possible - but if you really need something sweet, then add a small amount of it (make sure to buy pure stevia though)!

BREAKFAST

BONE BROTH BREAKFAST NOODLE SOUP

Prep Time: 5 minutes
Cook Time: 10 minutes
Total Time: 15 minutes
Yield: 2 servings
Serving Size: 1 bowl

In Vietnam, breakfast is often noodles in bone broth for breakfast! So this is a keto version of that.

INGREDIENTS

- 4 cups *(960 ml)* of bone broth or chicken broth
- 1 zucchini, shredded
- 1 lime, juiced
- 1/2 teaspoon *(1 g)* fresh ginger, grated
- 1/2 teaspoon *(1 g)* cinnamon
- 1 Tablespoon *(2 g)* cilantro (or basil leaves), chopped

INSTRUCTIONS

1. Bring the chicken broth to a boil.
2. Add in the lime juice, grated ginger, cinnamon, and then the zucchini.
3. Boil for 2 minutes.
4. Add in the cilantro and serve.

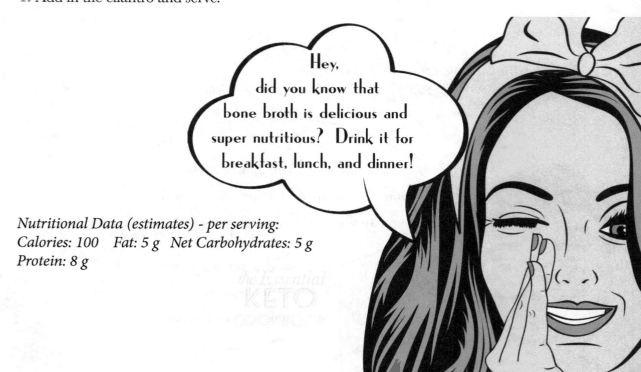

Hey, did you know that bone broth is delicious and super nutritious? Drink it for breakfast, lunch, and dinner!

Nutritional Data (estimates) - per serving:
Calories: 100   Fat: 5 g   Net Carbohydrates: 5 g
Protein: 8 g

EASY SEED & NUT GRANOLA

Prep Time: 5 minutes
Cook Time: 0 minutes
Total Time: 5 minutes
Yield: 1 serving
Serving Size: 1 bowl

INGREDIENTS

- 10 whole almonds
- 3 Brazil nuts
- 5 cashews
- 2 Tablespoons *(17 g)* pumpkin seeds
- 1 teaspoon *(3 g)* chia seeds
- 1 Tablespoon *(12 g)* cacao nibs
- 1 Tablespoon *(5 g)* coconut flakes
- 1/4 cup *(60 ml)* coconut milk

You can make these in advance and store in an airtight container for easy and fast breakfasts and snacks.

INSTRUCTIONS

1. Mix together all the dry ingredients. If you're making a large batch, then store leftovers in an airtight container.
2. Serve with coconut milk.

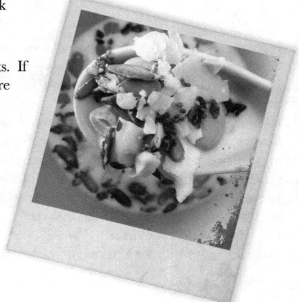

Nutritional Data (estimates) - per serving:
Calories: 400   Fat: 30 g   Net Carbohydrates: 9 g   Protein: 9 g

BREAKFAST

SPRING SOUP WITH POACHED EGG

Prep Time: 5 minutes
Cook Time: 15 minutes
Total Time: 20 minutes
Yield: 2 servings
Serving Size: 1 bowl

You can obviously make poached eggs and serve them over some cooked vegetables (like asparagus), but try the poached egg in broth for some variety.

INGREDIENTS

- 2 eggs
- 2 teaspoons *(10 ml)* of apple cider vinegar
- 32 oz *(1 l)* chicken broth (or bone broth)
- 1 head of romaine lettuce, chopped (or other leafy green vegetables)
- Salt to taste

INSTRUCTIONS

1. Place the chicken broth and apple cider vinegar into a pot and bring to a boil.
2. Crack an egg into a bowl and turn down the heat on the pot.
3. Use a spoon to start stirring the broth in the pan to create a whirlpool (i.e., stir in a circle).
4. Drop the eggs into the pot while the broth is still spinning.
5. Leave to cook on a medium heat so that the broth isn't boiling. For a soft but not runny poached egg, cook in the water for 5 minutes. If you prefer a runny poached egg, then remove from the water after around 3 minutes.
6. Remove the eggs and place one into each bowl.
7. Add the chopped romaine lettuce into the broth and cook for a few minutes until slightly wilted. Add salt to taste.
8. Ladle the broth with the lettuce into the bowls.

Nutritional Data (estimates) - per serving:
Calories: 150   Fat: 5 g   Net Carbohydrates: 4 g   Protein: 16 g

SPINACH, MUSHROOM, BACON SAUTE

Prep Time: 10 minutes
Cook Time: 10 minutes
Total Time: 20 minutes
Yield: 2 servings
Serving Size: 1 plate

Who says sautes aren't for breakfast! This is a simple egg-free recipe that you can enjoy at any time of the day. It's also a great way to get more spinach into your diet.

INGREDIENTS

- 4 slices of bacon, chopped
- 1/4 onion, chopped
- 3 button mushrooms, chopped
- 1 lb (*454 g*) spinach
- Salt to taste

INSTRUCTIONS

1. Add the chopped bacon into a saute pan.
2. After some of the fat has come out of the bacon, add the chopped onions into the pan and cook until the bacon is cooked and the onions are translucent.
3. Then add in the chopped mushrooms and lastly the spinach leaves.
4. Cook until spinach wilts. Add salt to taste and serve.

Nutritional Data (estimates) - per serving:
Calories: 130   Fat: 8 g   Net Carbohydrates: 4 g   Protein: 9 g

the Essential
KETO

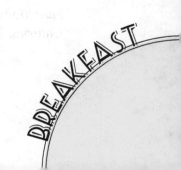

BREAKFAST

TEA EGGS (CHA DAN)

Prep Time: 15 minutes
Cook Time: 4 hours
Total Time: 4 hours 15 minutes
Yield: 6 servings
Serving Size: 2 eggs

Make a large batch of these tea eggs and enjoy for breakfast over several days. They also make great snacks during the day.

INGREDIENTS

- 12 eggs
- 2-4 black tea bags (depends how strong the tea is and how strong you want the flavor to be)
- 2 Tablespoons *(30 g)* salt
- 1/4 cup *(60 ml)* tamari sauce
- 2 Tablespoons *(14 g)* cinnamon powder
- 20 Szechuan peppercorns (or use regular peppercorns)
- 6 star anise
- 1 teaspoon *(2 g)* black pepper
- 6-8 cups *(1.5 - 2 l)* water

INSTRUCTIONS

1. Hard boil the eggs in water.
2. After the eggs are hard boiled, cool the eggs and crack the shell so that the shell is still intact but very cracked.
3. Add the tea bags, salt, tamari sauce, cinnamon, Szechuan peppercorns, star anise, and black pepper into a large pot.
4. Add the cracked boiled eggs into the pot.
5. Add 6-8 cups of water to the pot (ensuring the eggs are covered).
6. Simmer on a low heat with the lid on.
7. Remove the tea bags after 30 minutes.
8. Continue simmering with the lid on for 3.5 more hours.
9. Cool the eggs and remove the shell.

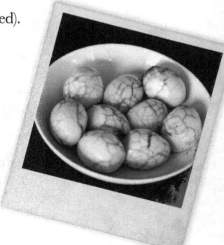

Nutritional Data (estimates) - per serving:
Calories: 140   Fat: 9 g   Net Carbohydrates: 1 g   Protein: 12 g

the Essential
KETO

BREAKFAST GREEN SMOOTHIE

Prep Time: 5 minutes
Cook Time: 0 minutes
Total Time: 5 minutes
Yield: 1 serving
Serving Size: 1 cup

Psyllium seeds are a great source of soluble dietary fiber - it'll help keep your gut bacteria functioning well. If you have trouble finding them, then you can omit it from the recipe.

INGREDIENTS

- 2 cups *(60 g)* spinach (or other leafy greens)
- ⅓ cup *(46 g)* raw almonds
- 2 Brazil nuts
- 1 cup *(240 ml)* coconut milk (unsweetened - from refrigerated cartons not cans)
- 1 scoop *(~20 g)* greens powder (optional)
- 1 Tablespoon *(10 g)* psyllium seeds (or psyllium husks) or chia seeds

INSTRUCTIONS

1. Place the spinach, almonds, Brazil nuts, and coconut milk into the blender first.
2. Blend until pureed.
3. Add in the rest of the ingredients (greens powder, psyllium seeds) and blend well.

Nutritional Data (estimates) - per serving:
Calories: 380   Fat: 30 g   Net Carbohydrates: 5 g   Protein: 12 g

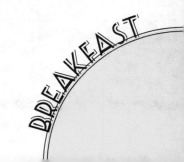

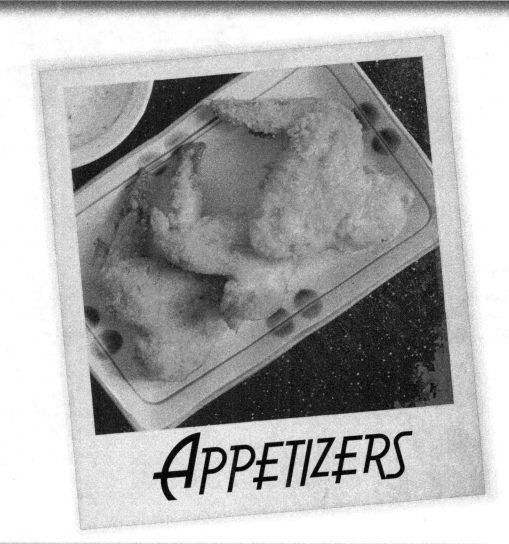

APPETIZERS

CHAPTER 2

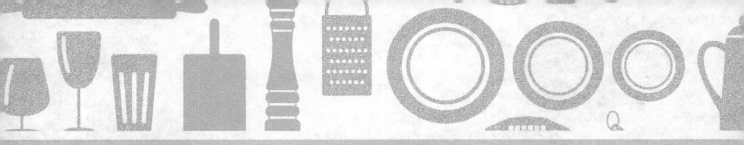

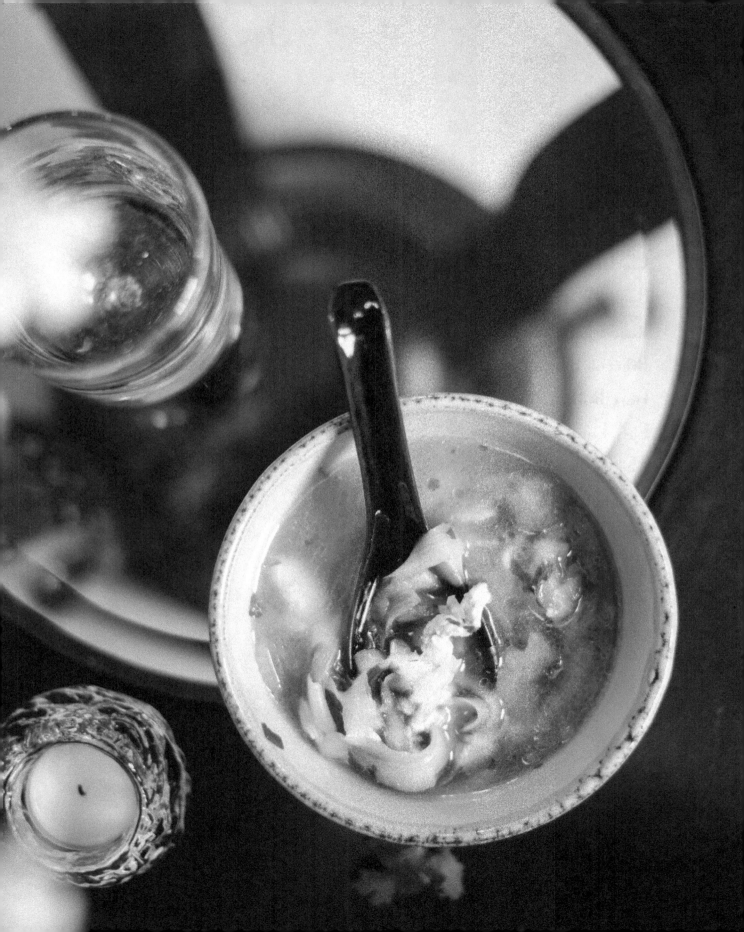

CHICKEN NOODLE SOUP

Prep Time: 15 minutes
Cook Time: 15 minutes
Total Time: 30 minutes
Yield: 2 servings
Serving Size: 1 large bowl

INGREDIENTS

- 3 cups *(720 ml)* chicken broth or bone broth
- 1 chicken breast *(approx 225 g or 0.5 lb)*, chopped into small pieces
- 2 Tablespoons *(30 ml)* avocado oil
- 1 stalk of celery, chopped
- 1 green onion, chopped
- 1/4 cup *(8 g)* cilantro, finely chopped
- 1 zucchini, peeled
- Salt to taste

INSTRUCTIONS

1. Add the avocado oil into a saucepan and saute the diced chicken in there until cooked.
2. Add chicken broth to the same saucepan and simmer.
3. Add the chopped celery and green onion into the saucepan.
4. Create zucchini noodles – I used a potato peeler to create long strands, but other options include using a spiralizer or a food processor with the shredding attachment.
5. Add zucchini noodles and finely chopped cilantro to the saucepan. Simmer for a few more minutes, add salt to taste, and serve immediately.

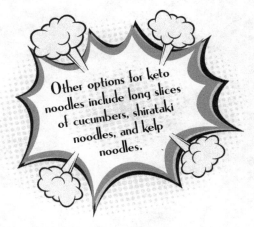

Other options for keto noodles include long slices of cucumbers, shirataki noodles, and kelp noodles.

Nutritional Data (estimates) - per serving:
Calories: 310   Fat: 16 g   Net Carbohydrates: 4 g   Protein: 34 g

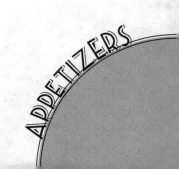

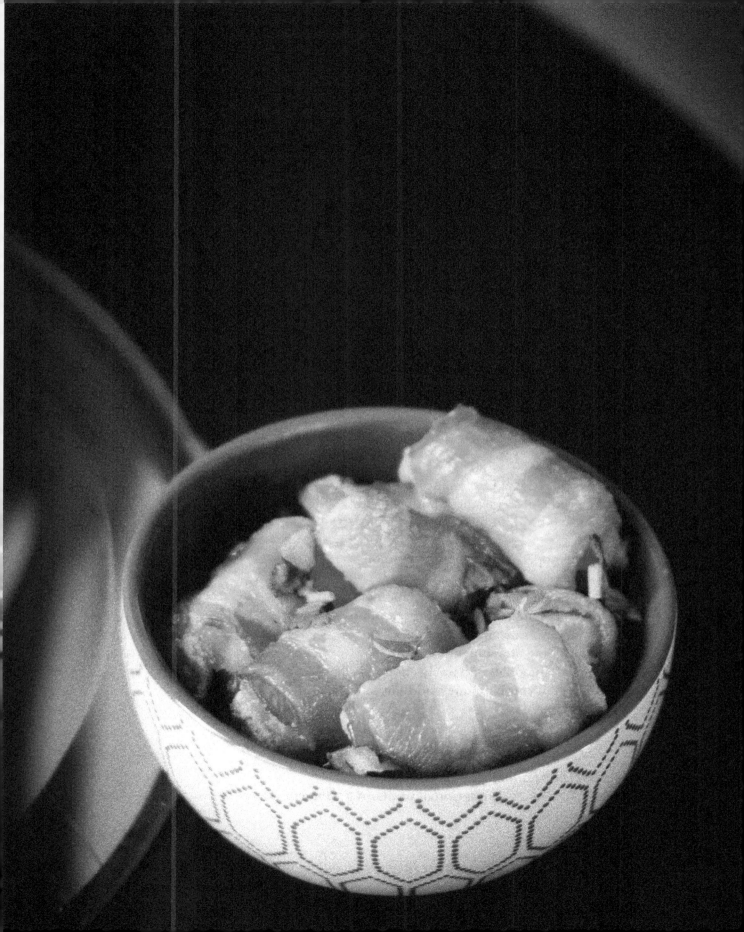

BACON WRAPPED CHICKEN BITES WITH GARLIC MAYO

Prep Time: 10 minutes
Cook Time: 30 minutes
Total Time: 40 minutes
Yield: 4 servings
Serving Size: 6 bites

INGREDIENTS

- 1 large chicken breast *(approx 225 g or 0.5 lb)*, cut into small bites (approx. 22-27 pieces)
- 8-9 thin slices of bacon, cut into thirds
- 3 Tablespoons *(30 g)* garlic powder

For the garlic mayo:

- 1/4 cup *(60 ml)* mayo (see page 181 for recipe)
- 2 cloves of garlic, minced
- Dash of salt
- Dash of chili powder (optional)
- 1 teaspoon *(5 ml)* lemon juice (optional)
- 1 teaspoon *(4 g)* garlic powder (optional)

INSTRUCTIONS

1. Preheat oven to 400 F *(200 C)* and line a baking tray with foil.
2. Place the garlic power into a small bowl and dip each small chunk of chicken in it.
3. Wrap each short bacon piece around each garlic powder-dipped piece of chicken. Place the bacon wrapped chicken bites on the baking tray. (Try to space them out so they're not touching on the tray.)
4. Bake for 25-30 minutes until the bacon turns crispy.
5. Meanwhile, combine the garlic mayo ingredients in a small bowl and use a fork to whisk it slightly.
6. Serve the bacon wrapped chicken bites with cocktail sticks and the garlic mayo.

Nutritional Data (estimates) - per serving:
Calories: 350   Fat: 27 g   Net Carbohydrates: 5 g   Protein: 22 g

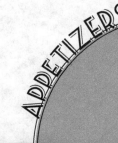

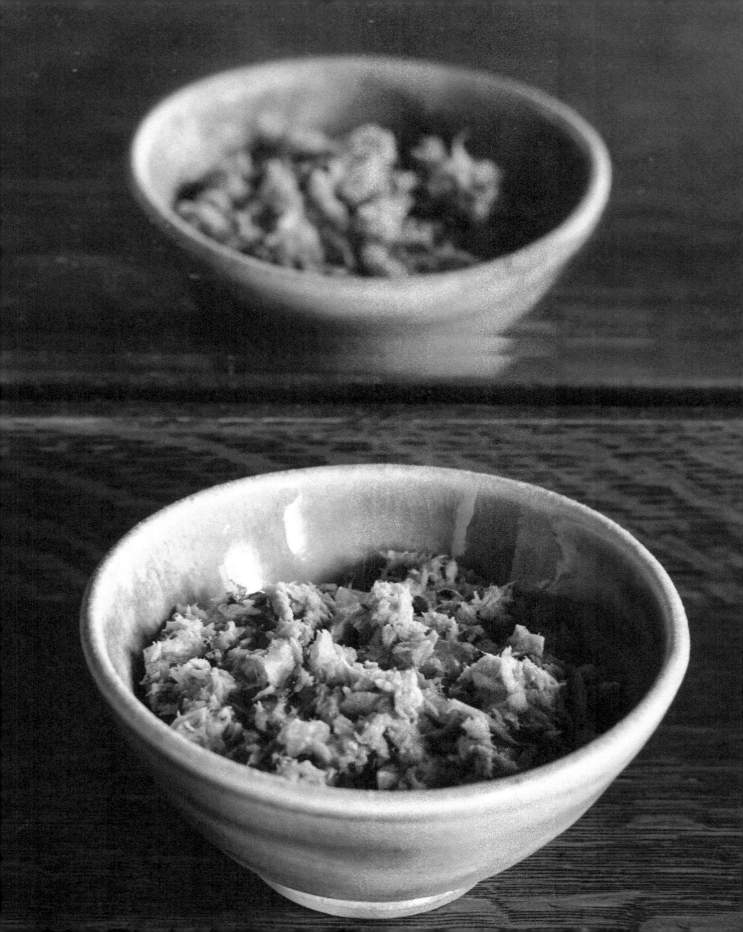

ITALIAN TUNA SALAD

Prep Time: 10 minutes
Cook Time: 0 minutes
Total Time: 10 minutes
Yield: 2 servings
Serving Size: 1 cup

INGREDIENTS

- 10 cherry tomatoes (or 5 sun-dried tomatoes)
- 2 *(5 oz or 140 g)* cans of tuna
- 1-2 ribs of celery, finely diced
- 1 clove of garlic, minced
- 3 Tablespoons *(6 g)* parsley, finely chopped
- 1/2 Tablespoon *(7 ml)* lemon juice
- 2 Tablespoons *(30 ml)* olive oil
- Salt and pepper to taste

INSTRUCTIONS

1. Halve the cherry tomatoes (if you're using sun-dried tomatoes, you may need to soak them first).
2. Flake the tuna.
3. Mix all ingredients together in a bowl and serve.

SUBSTITUTIONS

- Cucumbers can be used instead of the tomatoes.

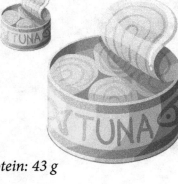

Nutritional Data (estimates) - per serving:
Calories: 330   Fat: 15 g   Net Carbohydrates: 3 g   Protein: 43 g

APPETIZERS

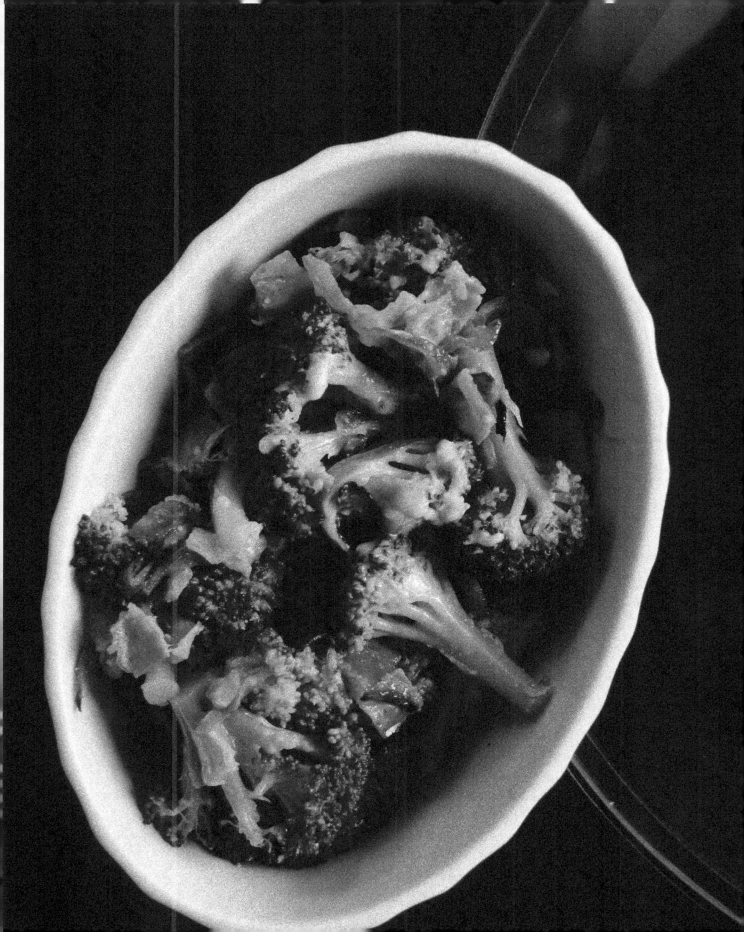

BROCCOLI BACON SALAD

Prep Time: 10 minutes
Cook Time: 30 minutes
Total Time: 40 minutes
Yield: 6 servings
Serving Size: 1 bowl

INGREDIENTS

- 1 lb *(454 g)* broccoli florets
- 4 small red onions or 2 large ones, sliced
- 20 slices of bacon, chopped into small pieces
- 1 cup *(240 ml)* coconut milk
    or 1/2 cup *(120 ml)* coconut ranch dressing (see page 182 for recipe)
- Salt to taste

INSTRUCTIONS

1. Cook the bacon first, and then cook the onions in the bacon fat.
2. Blanche the broccoli florets (or you can use them raw or soften them by boiling them first).
3. Toss the bacon pieces, onions, and broccoli florets together with the coconut milk and salt to taste.
4. Serve at room temperature.

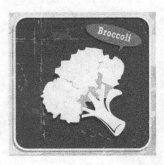

Nutritional Data (estimates) - per serving:
Calories: 280   Fat: 26 g   Net Carbohydrates: 5 g   Protein: 7 g

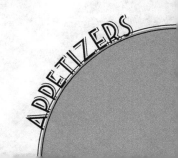

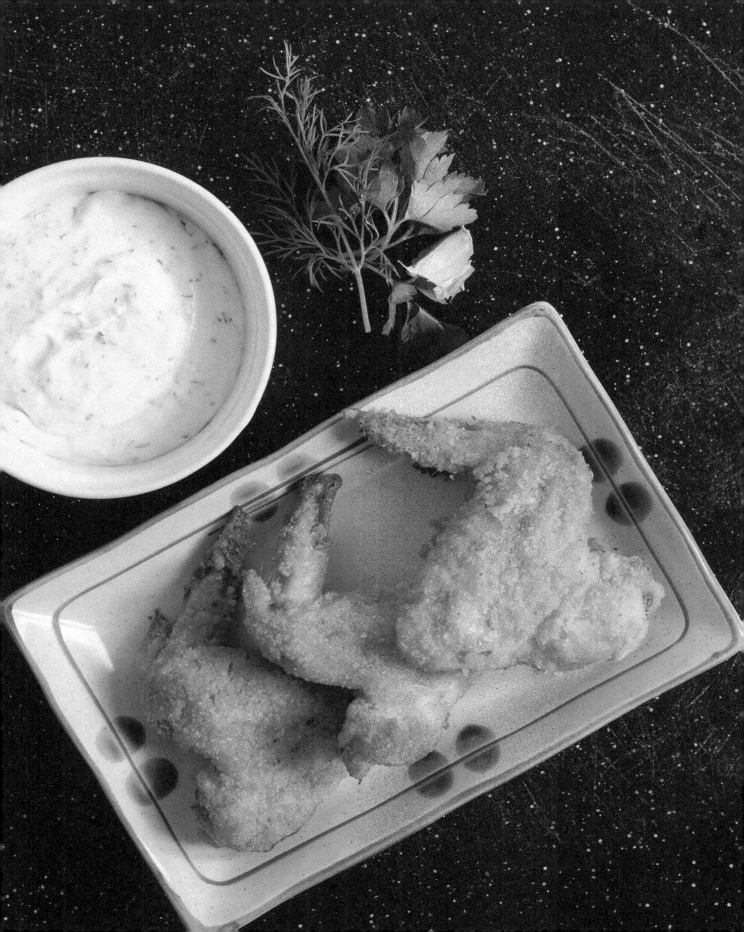

FIERY BUFFALO WINGS

Prep Time: 15 minutes
Cook Time: 45 minutes
Total Time: 1 hour
Yield: 4 servings
Serving Size: 3 wings

INGREDIENTS

- 12 small chicken wings
- 1/2 cup *(56 g)* coconut flour
- 1/2 teaspoon *(1 g)* cayenne pepper
- 1/2 teaspoon *(1 g)* black pepper
- 1/2 teaspoon *(1 g)* crushed red pepper flakes
- 1 Tablespoon *(7 g)* paprika
- 1 Tablespoon *(8 g)* garlic powder
- 1 Tablespoon *(15 g)* salt
- 1/4 cup *(60 ml)* ghee, melted
- 1/4 cup *(60 ml)* hot sauce

INSTRUCTIONS

1. Preheat oven to 400 F *(200 C)*.
2. Mix the coconut flour, dried spices, and salt together in a bowl.
3. Coat each chicken wing with the coconut flour mixture. Refrigerate for 15-30 minutes to help the flour stick a bit better to the wings *(optional)*.
4. Grease a baking tray *(or line it with aluminum foil)*.
5. Mix the ghee and the hot sauce together well.
6. Dip each chicken wing into the ghee and hot sauce mixture and place onto the baking tray.
7. Bake for 45 minutes.

SUBSTITUTIONS

- If you omit any spices, increase the amount of garlic powder.

Nutritional Data (estimates) - per serving:
Calories: 500   Fat: 38 g   Net Carbohydrates: 3 g   Protein: 29 g

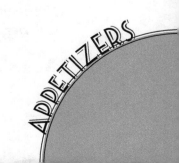

EASY EGG DROP SOUP

Prep Time: 5 minutes
Cook Time: 10 minutes
Total Time: 15 minutes
Yield: 1 serving
Serving Size: 1 large bowl

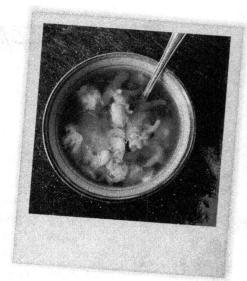

INGREDIENTS

- 2 cups *(480 ml)* chicken broth or bone broth
- 1/4 cup *(17 g)* scallions (chopped green onions)
- 1/2 tomato, sliced
- 1 egg, whisked
- 1 Tablespoon *(15 ml)* tamari sauce
- 1/2 teaspoon *(1 g)* fresh ginger, grated (optional)
- Salt and pepper to taste

INSTRUCTIONS

1. Heat up the chicken broth *(or other broth)* in a saucepan.
2. Slowly drizzle in the whisked egg while stirring slowly clockwise until the ribbons form.
3. Add the scallions, tomato, tamari sauce, grated ginger, salt, and pepper, and let it cook for a few minutes.

Nutritional Data (estimates) - per serving:
Calories: 130   Fat: 5 g   Net Carbohydrates: 5 g   Protein: 15 g

the Essential
KETO

THAI LEMONGRASS SHRIMP SOUP

Prep Time: 10 minutes
Cook Time: 30 minutes
Total Time: 40 minutes
Yield: 4 servings
Serving Size: 1 bowl

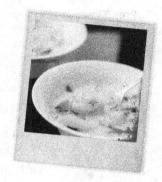

INGREDIENTS

- 16 large shrimp *(approx. 1 lb (454 g))*
- 1 cup *(240 ml)* coconut cream *(top layer of cream from a refrigerated can of coconut milk)*
- 1 quart *(950 ml)* chicken broth or bone broth
- 3 large button mushrooms, sliced
- 1 lemongrass stalk, split down the center and chopped into 2-inch chunks
- 1 teaspoon *(2 g)* ginger, freshly grated *(traditional recipe uses thin slices of galangal)*
- 1 small Thai chili (optional), finely diced
- 3 Tablespoons *(45 ml)* fish sauce
- Juice of 1/2 of a lime
- Salt to taste
- 2 Tablespoons *(4 g)* cilantro, finely chopped *(for garnish)*

INSTRUCTIONS

1. Heat the chicken broth in a medium-sized pot and add in the mushrooms, lemongrass, ginger, chili, fish sauce, and lime juice.
2. Simmer for 10 minutes.
3. Add in the coconut cream and simmer for another 10 minutes until the coconut cream mixes in well.
4. Taste the broth and add in salt to taste. Add in more fish sauce, lime juice, or coconut cream depending on how you like the soup.
5. Add in the shrimp and simmer for 8-10 minutes.
6. Serve immediately with the cilantro as garnish.

Nutritional Data (estimates) - per serving:
Calories: 340   Fat: 23 g   Net Carbohydrates: 5 g   Protein: 29 g

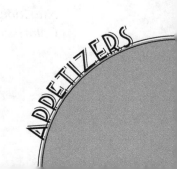

APPETIZERS

SPAGHETTI SQUASH SOUP

Prep Time: 15 minutes
Cook Time: 25 minutes
Total Time: 40 minutes
Yield: 4 servings
Serving Size: 1 cup

INGREDIENTS

- 1 spaghetti squash
- 2 cups *(480 ml)* chicken broth or bone broth
- 2 teaspoons *(4 g)* cinnamon
- Dash of nutmeg
- Dash of cloves
- 1 Tablespoon *(15 ml)* apple cider vinegar
- Salt and pepper to taste

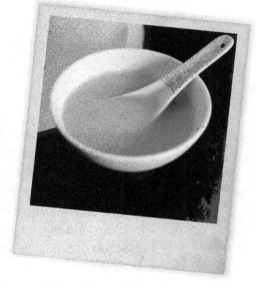

INSTRUCTIONS

1. Pour the chicken broth into a large pot on medium heat. Cut the spaghetti squash into chunks (removing the outer skin and the seeds) and place into the pot. Cook until the squash is very tender.
2. Use an immersion blender to puree the squash. (If you don't have an immersion blender, then just remove the squash pieces and puree in a blender or food processor and then pour back into the pot.)
3. Mix in the cinnamon, nutmeg, cloves, apple cider vinegar, salt, and pepper to taste.

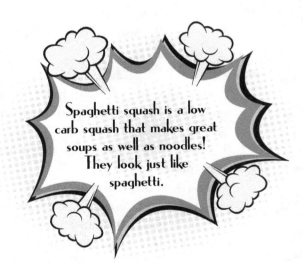

Spaghetti squash is a low carb squash that makes great soups as well as noodles! They look just like spaghetti.

Nutritional Data (estimates) - per serving:
Calories: 50   Fat: 0 g   Net Carbohydrates: 5 g   Protein: 2 g

CRAB HASH WITH GINGER AND CILANTRO

Prep Time: 10 minutes
Cook Time: 15 minutes
Total Time: 25 minutes
Yield: 4-6 servings
Serving Size: 1 small plate

INGREDIENTS

- 2 zucchinis, peeled and shredded
- 1 lb *(454 g)* lump crabmeat *(fresh or canned)*
- 1/4 cup *(17 g)* scallions (green onions) chopped (optional)
- 1/4 cup *(8 g)* cilantro, finely chopped
- 2 cloves of garlic, minced
- 2 teaspoons *(4 g)* fresh ginger, grated
- 1 Tablespoon *(15 ml)* lemon juice
- 2 boiled eggs, diced (optional)
- Salt to taste
- 2 Tablespoons *(30 ml)* coconut oil

INSTRUCTIONS

1. Place 2 Tablespoons of coconut oil into a frying pan *(or a saucepan)*.
2. Add in the shredded zucchinis, crabmeat, and scallions and sauté for 5-10 minutes.
3. Lastly, add the cilantro, garlic, ginger, lemon juice, and salt to taste. Sauté for a few minutes more to combine the flavors.
4. Top with the diced boiled eggs (optional) and serve immediately.

SUBSTITUTIONS

- Chicken breast *(finely diced)* can be used instead of crabmeat, but you should cook it separately first.
- Scrambled eggs can be used instead of boiled eggs.
- Apple cider vinegar can be used instead of lemon juice.

Nutritional Data (estimates) - per serving:
Calories: 150   Fat: 7 g   Net Carbohydrates: 2 g   Protein: 19 g

APPETIZERS

HEARTY CAULIFLOWER, LEEK & BACON SOUP

Prep Time: 10 minutes
Cook Time: 1 hour
Total Time: 1 hour 10 minutes
Yield: 4 servings
Serving Size: 1 cup

INGREDIENTS

- 1/2 head of cauliflower, chopped
- 6 cups *(1.4 l)* chicken broth or bone broth
- 1 leek, chopped
- 5 slices of bacon, cooked
- Salt and pepper to taste

INSTRUCTIONS

1. Place the chopped cauliflower and leek into a pot with the chicken broth.
2. Cover the pot and simmer for 1 hour or until tender.
3. Use an immersion blender to puree the vegetables to create a smooth soup. *(If you don't have an immersion blender, you can take the vegetables out, let cool briefly, puree in a normal blender, and then put back into the pot.)*
4. Crumble the cooked bacon into small pieces and drop into the soup.
5. Add salt and pepper to taste.

SUBSTITUTIONS

- Onion can be used instead of leek *(use 1 small white or yellow onion)*.

Nutritional Data (estimates) - per serving:
Calories: 110   Fat: 4 g   Net Carbohydrates: 6 g   Protein: 10 g

BIG EASY SALAD

Prep Time: 15 minutes
Cook Time: 0 minutes
Total Time: 15 minutes
Yield: 2 servings
Serving Size: 1 large bowl or plate

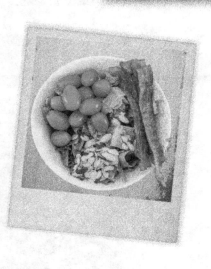

INGREDIENTS

- 2 romaine lettuce, chopped into small pieces
- 10 cherry or grape tomatoes
- 1 Tablespoon *(4 g)* sliced almonds (optional)
- 4-6 slices of bacon, cooked (crumbled)
- 1/2 lb *(225 g)* ham, diced
- Olive oil and balsamic vinegar (or lemon juice) as dressing
    (or pick a dressing from the condiment recipes section)

INSTRUCTIONS

1. Add all the ingredients together and toss with olive oil and small amount of balsamic vinegar to taste.

Nutritional Data (estimates) - per serving:
Calories: 570   Fat: 36 g   Net Carbohydrates: 10 g   Protein: 40 g

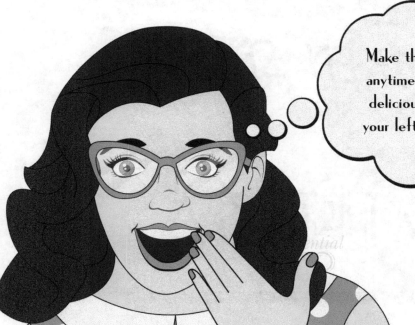

Make this big easy salad anytime for a super fast, delicious meal! Toss all your leftover veggies and meats in.

APPETIZERS

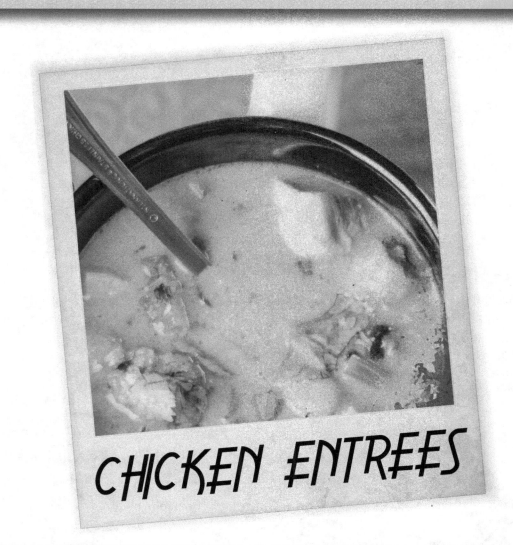

CHICKEN ENTREES

CHAPTER 3A

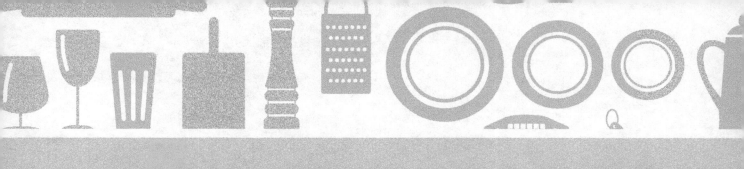

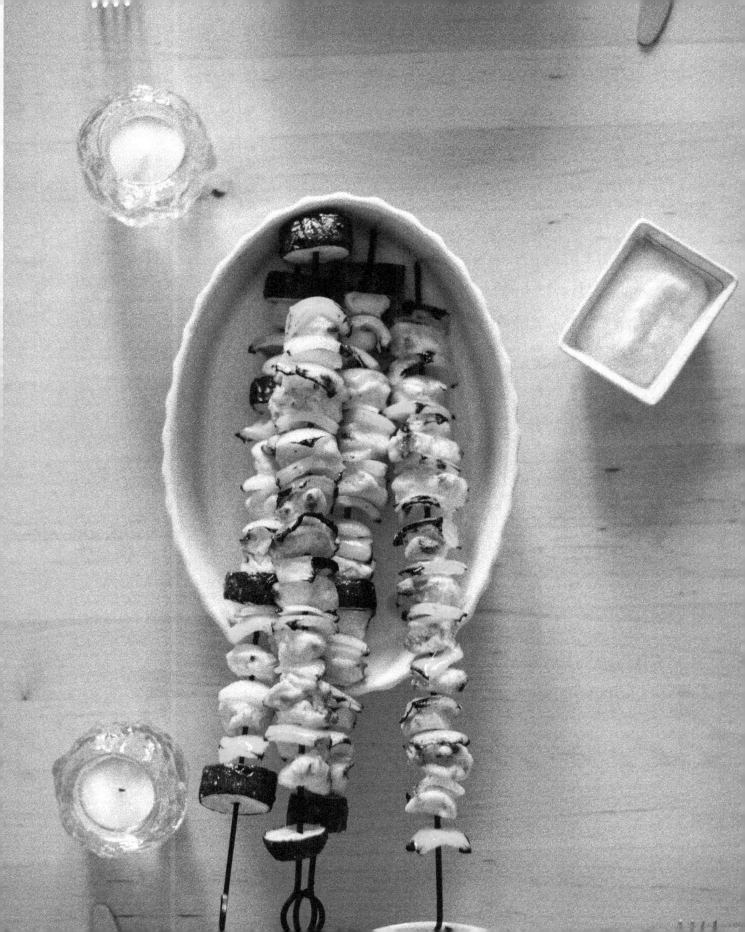

GRILLED CHICKEN SKEWERS WITH GARLIC SAUCE

Prep Time: 15 minutes
Cook Time: 15 minutes
Total Time: 30 minutes
Yield: 2 servings
Serving Size: 2 skewers

INGREDIENTS

For the skewers:
- 1 lb *(454 g)* chicken breast, cut into large cubes (approx 1-inch)
- 1 onion, chopped
- 2 bell peppers, chopped
- 1 zucchini

For the garlic sauce:
- 1 head of garlic, peeled
- 1 teaspoon *(5 g)* salt
- Approx. 1/4 cup *(60 ml)* lemon juice
- Approx. 1 cup *(240 ml)* olive oil

For the marinade:
- 1/2 cup *(120 ml)* olive oil
- 1 teaspoon *(5 g)* salt

INSTRUCTIONS

1. Heat up the grill to high. If using wooden skewers, soak them in water first.
2. For the garlic sauce, place the garlic cloves and salt into the blender. Then add in around 1/8 cup of the lemon juice and 1/2 cup of olive oil.
3. Blend well for 5-10 seconds, then slow your blender down and drizzle in more lemon juice and olive oil alternatively until it forms a smooth consistency.
4. Keep half the garlic sauce to serve with.
5. Take the other half of the garlic sauce and add in the additional 1/2 cup of olive oil and teaspoon of salt. Mix well - this makes the marinade.
6. Chop the chicken, onion, bell peppers, and zucchini into approximate 1-inch cubes or squares. Mix them in a bowl with the marinade.
7. Place the cubes on skewers and grill on high until the chicken is cooked (usually, we grill on the bottom for a few minutes to get the charred look and then move the skewers to a top rack with the lid down to cook the chicken well).
8. Serve with the garlic sauce you kept.

Nutritional Data (estimates) - per serving:
Calories: 580   Fat: 33 g   Net Carbohydrates: 9 g   Protein: 55 g

CHICKEN

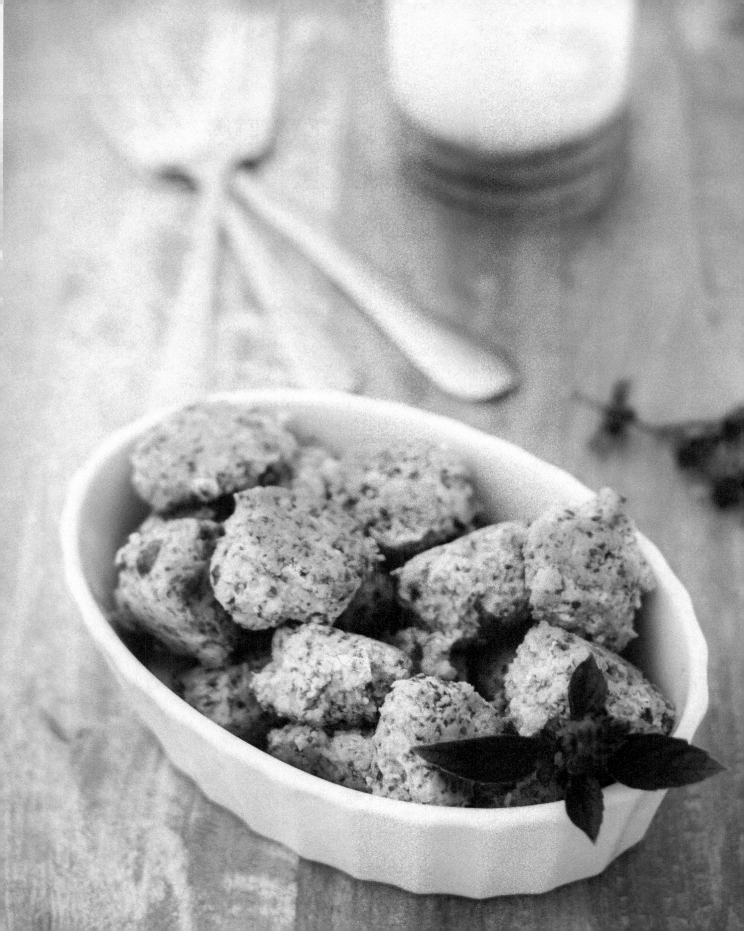

SPINACH BASIL CHICKEN MEATBALLS

Prep Time: 10 minutes
Cook Time: 15 minutes
Total Time: 25 minutes
Yield: 2 servings
Serving Size: 10-12 meatballs

INGREDIENTS

- 2 chicken breasts *(approx. 1 lb or 454 g)*
- 1/4 lb *(115 g)* spinach
- 2 teaspoons *(10 g)* salt
- 10 basil leaves
- 5 cloves of garlic, peeled
- 3 Tablespoons *(45 ml)* olive oil
- 2 Tablespoons *(30 ml)* olive oil or avocado oil to cook in

INSTRUCTIONS

1. Place the chicken breasts, spinach, salt, basil leaves, garlic, and 3 Tablespoons of olive oil into a food processor and process well.

2. Make ping-pong sized meatballs from the meat mixture.

3. Add the 2 Tablespoons olive oil or avocado oil to a frying pan and fry the meatballs for 4 minutes on medium heat (fry in 2 batches if necessary). Turn the meatballs and fry for another 10 minutes. Make sure the meatballs don't get burnt.

4. Check the meatballs are fully cooked by cutting into one or using a meat thermometer.

> These are great as an appetizer or as an entree, and it's a fantastic way to get more spinach into your diet. Serve with some garlic sauce (see page 178 for recipe) or by themselves.

Nutritional Data (estimates) - per serving:
Calories: 600   Fat: 40 g   Net Carbohydrates: 4 g   Protein: 55 g

the Essential
KETO

CHICKEN

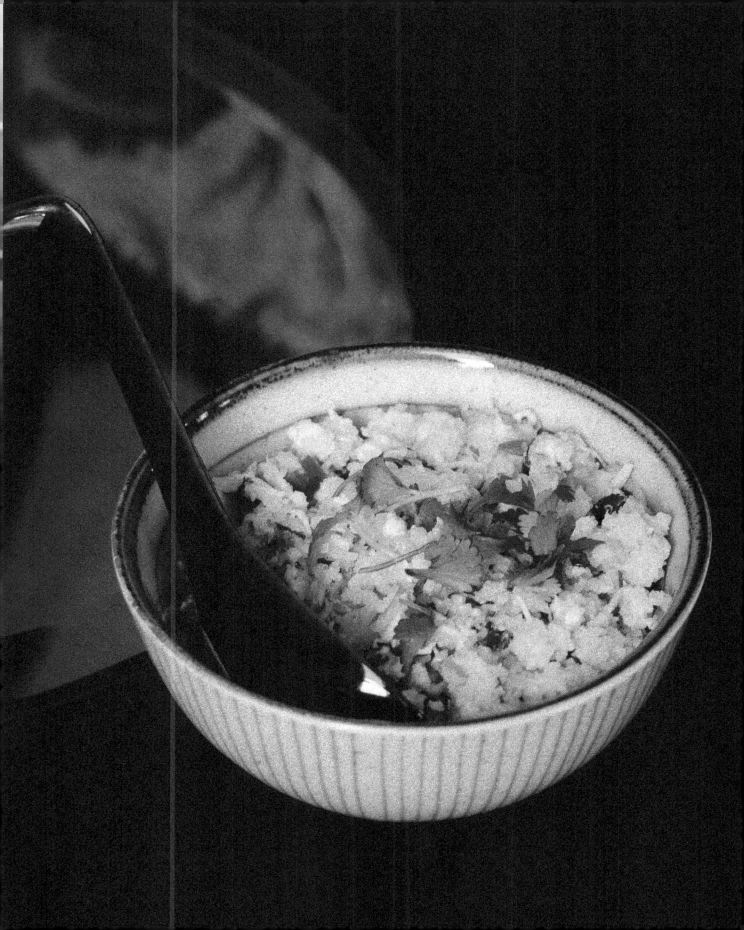

THAI CHICKEN AND "RICE"

Prep Time: 20 minutes
Cook Time: 20 minutes
Total Time: 40 minutes
Yield: 4 servings
Serving Size: 1 large bowl

You can make all sorts of cauliflower rice recipes - they're the perfect way to enjoy "rice" on a keto diet! Add some chopped chilis or a drizzle of Chinese chili oil (see page 185 for recipe) for a spicy version.

INGREDIENTS

- 1 head of cauliflower
- Meat from a whole roasted chicken (or use 3-4 cooked chicken breasts), shredded (or use some leftover meat)
- 2 eggs, whisked
- 1 Tablespoon *(5 g)* fresh ginger, grated
- 3 cloves of garlic, minced
- 1 Tablespoon *(15 ml)* tamari sauce
- 1/2 cup *(16 g)* cilantro, chopped
- Coconut oil to cook with
- Salt and pepper to taste

INSTRUCTIONS

1. If you don't have cooked shredded chicken, poach 3-4 chicken breasts and shred them or use another leftover meat.
2. Break the cauliflower into florets and food process until it forms a rice-like texture (may need to be done in batches). Squeeze excess water out.
3. Scramble 2 eggs in some coconut oil. Lightly salt the scrambled eggs and put aside while you make the cauliflower rice.
4. Place the cauliflower "rice" into a large pan with coconut oil and cook the cauliflower rice (may need to be done in 2 pans or in batches). Keep the heat on medium and stir regularly for 10 minutes.
5. Add in the shredded chicken, scrambled eggs, ginger, garlic, tamari sauce, cilantro, salt, and pepper to taste. Mix together, cook for another 2-3 minutes and serve.

Nutritional Data (estimates) - per serving:
Calories: 350   Fat: 11 g   Net Carbohydrates: 5 g   Protein: 55 g

the Essential
KETO

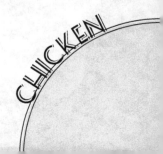
CHICKEN

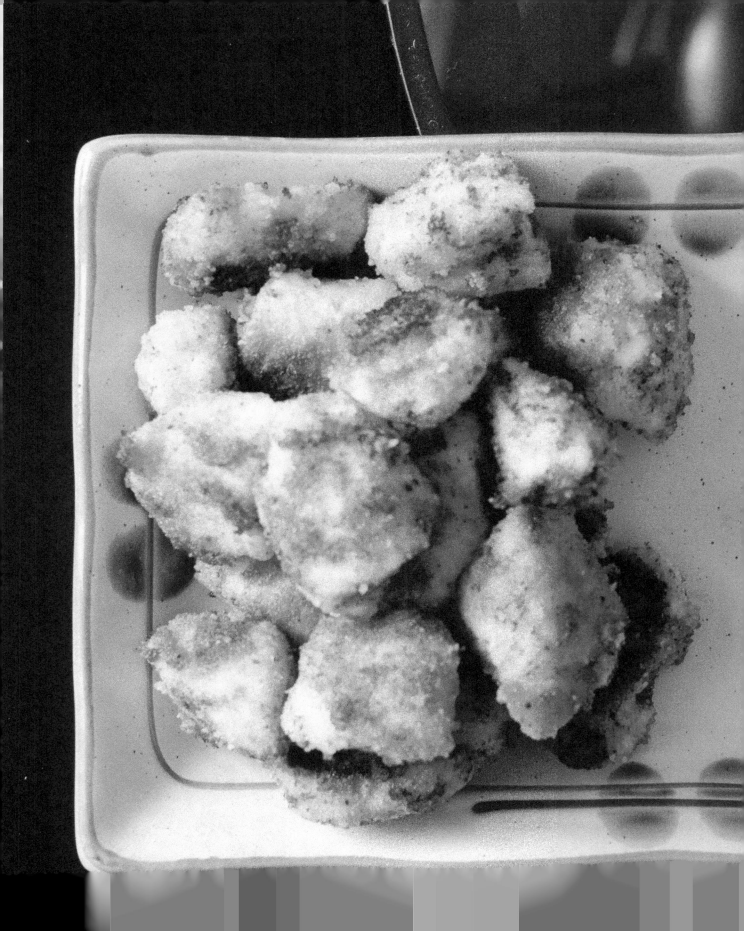

CHICKEN NUGGETS

Prep Time: 10 minutes
Cook Time: 15 minutes
Total Time: 25 minutes
Yield: 2 servings
Serving Size: 1 chicken breast

INGREDIENTS

- 2 chicken breasts, cut into cubes
- 1/2 cup *(56 g)* coconut flour
- 1 egg
- 2 Tablespoons *(20 g)* garlic powder
- 1 teaspoon *(5 g)* salt *(or to taste)*
- 1/4-1/2 cup *(60-120 ml)* ghee for shallow frying

INSTRUCTIONS

1. Cube the chicken breasts if you haven't done so already.
2. In a bowl, mix together the coconut flour, garlic powder, and salt. Taste the mixture to see if you'd like more salt.
3. In a separate bowl, whisk 1 egg to make the egg wash.
4. Place the ghee in a saucepan on medium heat *(or use a deep fryer)*.
5. Dip the cubed chicken in the egg wash and then drop into the coconut flour mixture to coat it with the "breading."
6. Carefully place some of the "breaded" chicken cubes into the ghee and fry until golden *(approx. 10 minutes)*. Make sure there's only a single layer of chicken in the pan so that they can all cook in the oil. Turn the chicken pieces to make sure they get cooked uniformly. Depending on the size of the pan, you might need to do this step in batches.
7. Place the cooked chicken pieces onto paper towels to soak up any excess oil. Enjoy by themselves or with some coconut ranch dressing (see page 182 for recipe) or garlic sauce (see page 178 for recipe).

Nutritional Data (estimates) - per serving:
Calories: 550   Fat: 27 g   Net Carbohydrates: 8 g   Protein: 60 g

CHICKEN

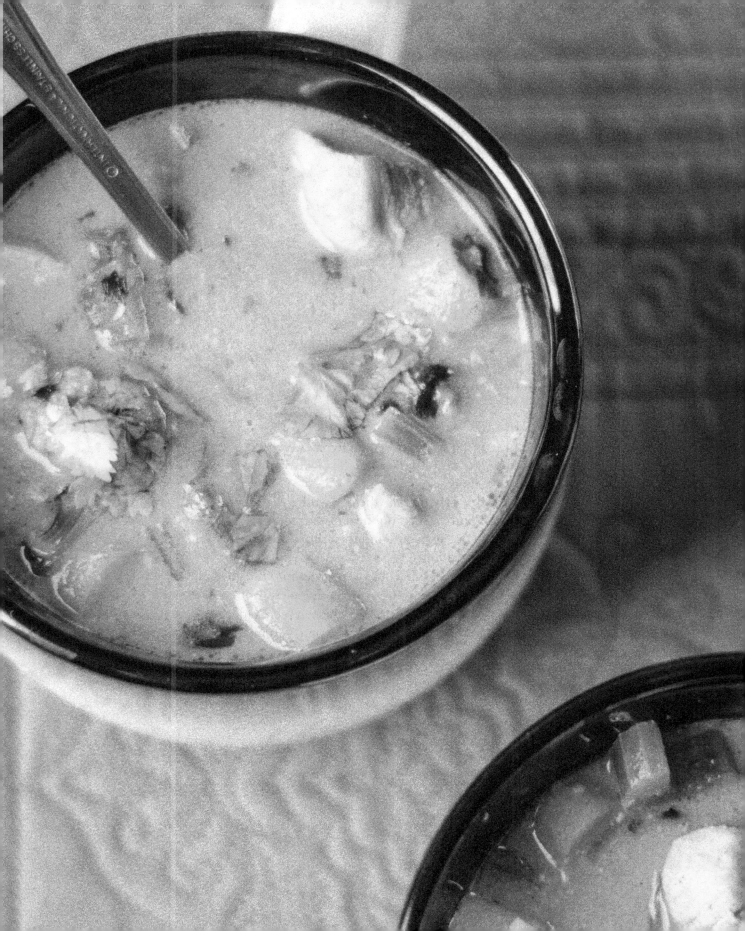

COCONUT CHICKEN CURRY

Prep Time: 15 minutes
Cook Time: 45 minutes
Total Time: 1 hour
Yield: 4 servings
Serving Size: 1 large bowl

Curries can be a delicious and very flavorful addition to your keto diet. This coconut chicken curry is an easy one to start with, but I encourage you to experiment!

INGREDIENTS

- 3 chicken breasts, cut into chunks
- 1 Tablespoon *(15 ml)* ghee or coconut oil
- 1 cup *(240 ml)* coconut cream (the top layer of cream from a refrigerated can of coconut milk)
- 1 cup *(240 ml)* chicken broth
- 2 cups *(250 g)* carrots (or zucchini), diced
- 1 cup *(100 g)* celery, chopped
- 2 tomatoes, diced
- 1 Tablespoon *(5 g)* fresh ginger, grated
- 1.5 Tablespoons *(10 g)* curry powder or garam masala
- 1/4 cup *(8 g)* cilantro, roughly chopped
- 6 cloves of garlic, minced
- Salt to taste

INSTRUCTIONS

1. Sauté the chicken in the ghee in a medium-sized saucepan.
2. When the outside of the chicken has all turned white, add in the coconut cream and the chicken broth and mix well.
3. Add in the carrots, celery, and tomatoes.
4. Add in the ginger and curry powder (or garam masala).
5. Cook on medium heat with the lid on for 40 minutes (stirring occasionally).
6. Add in the cilantro, minced garlic, and salt to taste. Cook for another 5 minutes and serve. Enjoy by itself, with a slice of Microwave Quick Bread (see page 141 for recipe), or with some Cauliflower White "Rice" (see page 143 for recipe).

Nutritional Data (estimates) - per serving:
Calories: 450   Fat: 25 g   Net Carbohydrates: 9 g   Protein: 45 g

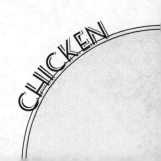

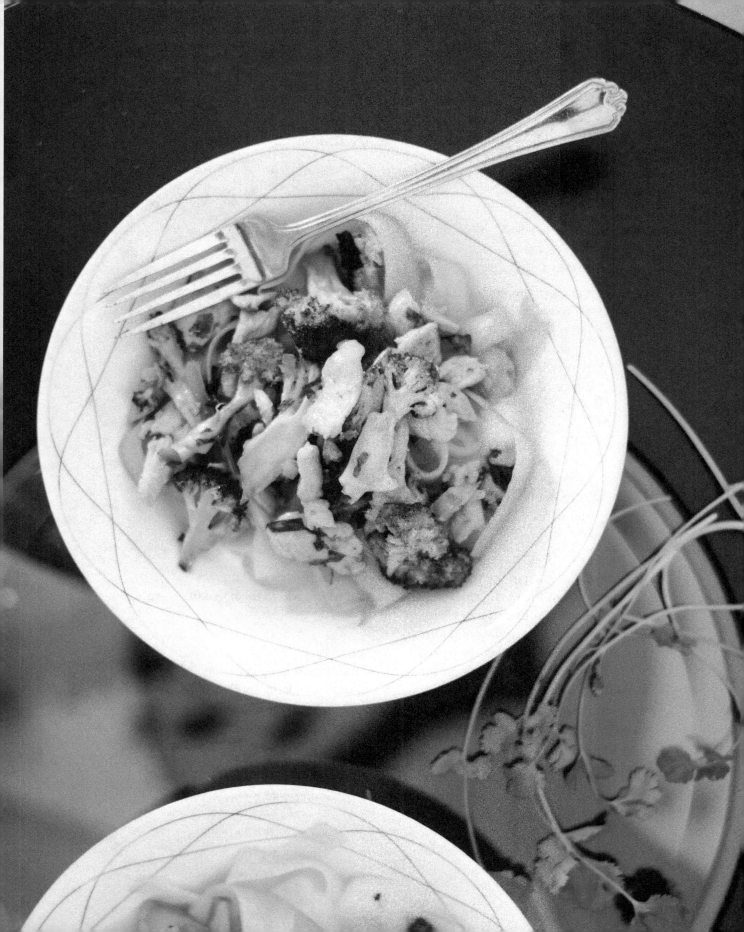

THAI CHICKEN PAD SEE EW

Prep Time: 10 minutes
Cook Time: 15 minutes
Total Time: 25 minutes
Yield: 2 servings
Serving Size: 1 large plate

Pad see ew is traditionally made with rice noodles, but this recipe uses cucumber noodles instead for a keto version of this delicious dish.

INGREDIENTS

- 1 chicken breast *(0.5 lb or 225 g)*, cut into small, thin pieces
- 1/4 cup *(17 g)* green onion, diced (scallions)
- 1 cup *(115 g)* broccoli, broken into small florets
- 1 teaspoon *(1 g)* fresh ginger, grated
- 1 Tablespoon *(15 ml)* tamari sauce
- 2 cloves of garlic, minced
- 1 Tablespoon *(2 g)* cilantro, finely chopped
- 1 Tablespoon *(15 ml)* coconut oil to cook in
- 1 cucumber, peeled into long noodles using a potato peeler
- Salt to taste

INSTRUCTIONS

1. Add 1 Tablespoon of coconut oil into a large saucepan and sauté the chicken breast and green onions in it.
2. Add in the broccoli, ginger, and tamari sauce. Place a lid over the saucepan and let the broccoli cook on medium heat until it's tender to your liking (approx. 5-10 minutes). Stir regularly.
3. Meanwhile, peel the cucumber and then create the cucumber noodles by using a potato peeler to peel the cucumber into long, wide strands. Divide the cucumber noodles between two plates.
4. Add to the saucepan the minced garlic, cilantro, and salt to taste. Serve on top of the cucumber noodles. Enjoy this entree with a bowl of the Thai Lemongrass Shrimp Soup (see page 53 for recipe) to start.

Nutritional Data (estimates) - per serving:
Calories: 280   Fat: 11 g   Net Carbohydrates: 5 g   Protein: 35 g

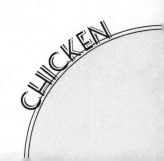

PRESSURE COOKER CHICKEN STEW

Prep Time: 15 minutes
Cook Time: 35 minutes
Total Time: 50 minutes
Yield: 3 servings
Serving Size: 1 bowl

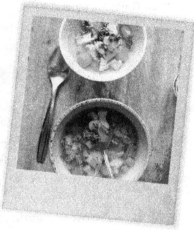

INGREDIENTS

- 2-3 chicken breasts *(approx. 1 lb or 454 g)*, diced
- 4 cups *(1 l)* chicken broth or bone broth
- 2 small carrots, chopped
- 3 stalks of celery, chopped
- 1/2 onion, chopped
- 1 teaspoon *(5 ml)* tamari sauce
- 1/2 Tablespoon *(1 g)* fresh thyme leaves *(or use 1/2 tsp (0.5 g) dried thyme)*
- 1/2 cup *(15 g)* parsley,
       chopped and divided (save half for when you're serving)
- 1 Tablespoon *(7 g)* unflavored gelatin powder (optional)
- Salt to taste

INSTRUCTIONS

1. Place the diced chicken breasts, chicken broth, chopped carrots, chopped celery, chopped onion, tamari sauce, thyme, and half the parsley into the pressure cooker pot.
2. If you're adding in gelatin, then stir it in until it dissolves.
3. Set the pressure cooker on high pressure for 35 minutes. When ready, follow your pressure cooker's instructions for releasing the pressure safely.
4. Add salt to taste and sprinkle in the rest of the chopped parsley.

Nutritional Data (estimates) - per serving:
Calories: 250   Fat: 4 g   Net Carbohydrates: 4 g   Protein: 44 g

CURRY GARLIC CRISPY CHICKEN DRUMSTICKS

Prep Time: 5 minutes
Cook Time: 40 minutes
Total Time: 45 minutes
Yield: 2 servings
Serving Size: 5 drumsticks

INGREDIENTS

- 10 chicken drumsticks
- 1-2 *(15-30 g)* Tablespoons salt
- 3 Tablespoons *(30 g)* curry powder
- 3 Tablespoons *(30 g)* garlic powder
- 1/2 Tablespoon *(7 ml)* of coconut oil for greasing baking tray (optional)

INSTRUCTIONS

1. Preheat oven to 450 F *(230 C)* and grease a large baking tray with coconut oil.
2. Mix the salt, curry powder, and garlic powder together in a bowl.
3. Coat each drumstick with the mixture, place on the baking tray, and bake for 40 minutes.

Nutritional Data (estimates) - per serving:
Calories: 630   Fat: 33 g   Net Carbohydrates: 4 g   Protein: 72 g

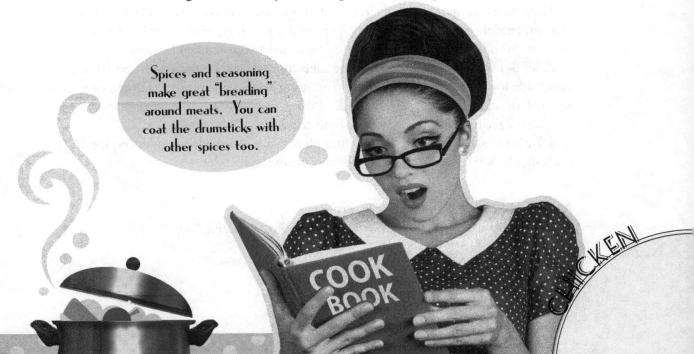

Spices and seasoning make great "breading" around meats. You can coat the drumsticks with other spices too.

CHICKEN

PAN-FRIED ITALIAN CHICKEN TENDERS

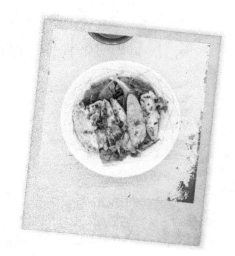

Prep Time: 15 minutes
Cook Time: 15 minutes
Total Time: 30 minutes
Yield: 2 servings
Serving Size: 6 chicken tenders

INGREDIENTS

- 1 lb *(454 g)* chicken tenders
    (approx. 12 chicken tenders)
- 2/3 cup *(160 ml)* olive oil + more for cooking
- 2 Tablespoons *(30 ml)* lime juice or white wine vinegar
- 1.5 Tablespoons *(20 g)* mustard
- 2 teaspoons *(2 g)* Italian seasoning (see page 177 for recipe)
- 4 cloves of garlic
- 1 teaspoon *(5 g)* salt and to taste
- Salad leaves

INSTRUCTIONS

1. Place the olive oil, lime juice or vinegar, mustard, Italian seasoning, garlic, and 1 teaspoon salt into the blender and blend well.

2. Heat up a frying pan and place 2 Tablespoons of olive oil into it. Place half the chicken tenders into the pan and cook on medium to high heat. Add in 1/3 of the mixture from the blender into the frying pan coating the chicken tenders.

3. After 3-4 minutes, flip the chicken tenders (they should be browned) and cook the other side for 2-3 minutes until done. Test using a meat thermometer or cut one open to see if the chicken is cooked through. Repeat for the rest of the chicken tenders (if you have 2 frying pans, you can cook both batches simultaneously).

4. Divide the salad between 2 plates and place 6 cooked chicken tenders on top of each salad. Serve with the rest of the sauce from the blender.

Nutritional Data (estimates) - per serving:
Calories: 600   Fat: 35 g   Net Carbohydrates: 3 g   Protein: 55 g

GRILLED CHICKEN DRUMSTICKS WITH GARLIC MARINADE

Prep Time: 10 minutes
Cook Time: 20 minutes
Total Time: 30 minutes
Yield: 2 servings
Serving Size: 3 drumsticks

INGREDIENTS

- 6 chicken drumsticks
- 1 cup *(240 ml)* olive oil
- 7 cloves of garlic
- 1 Tablespoon *(10 g)* garlic powder
- Juice from 1/2 lemon
- 1/2 Tablespoon *(7 g)* salt
- 1/2 teaspoon *(1 g)* pepper

INSTRUCTIONS

1. To make the marinade for the chicken, place the olive oil, garlic, garlic powder, lemon juice, salt, and pepper into a blender or food processor and puree.
2. Rub the chicken drumsticks in the marinade.
3. Grill the chicken drumsticks (use a low heat). Pour any leftover marinade over the chicken as it's grilling. If you need more sauce to serve with, make some of the garlic sauce (see page 178 for recipe).

Nutritional Data (estimates) - per serving:
Calories: 550   Fat: 42 g   Net Carbohydrates: 5 g   Protein: 43 g

the Essential
KETO

CHICKEN

SLOW COOKER BACON & CHICKEN

Prep Time: 10 minutes
Cook Time: 8 hours
Total Time: 8 hours 10 minutes
Yield: 6 servings
Serving Size: 1 plate

This is a really easy recipe, but it's absolutely delicious!

INGREDIENTS

- 5 chicken breasts
- 10 slices of bacon
- 2 Tablespoons *(9 g)* thyme *(dried)*
- 1 Tablespoon *(5 g)* oregano *(dried)*
- 1 Tablespoon *(3 g)* rosemary *(dried)*
- 5 Tablespoons *(75 ml)* olive oil *(2 Tbsp (30 ml) for the slow cooker and 3 Tbsp (45 ml) after cooking)*
- 1 Tablespoon *(15 g)* salt

INSTRUCTIONS

1. Place all the ingredients into a slow cooker pot and mix together.
2. Cook on the low temperature setting for 8 hours.
3. Shred the meat and mix with the 3 extra Tablespoons of olive oil.

SUBSTITUTIONS

• Italian seasoning (see page 177 for recipe) can be used instead of the thyme, oregano, and rosemary.

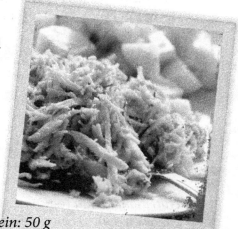

Nutritional Data (estimates) - per serving:
Calories: 580   Fat: 40 g   Net Carbohydrates: 0 g   Protein: 50 g

SLOW COOKER JERK CHICKEN

Prep Time: 10 minutes
Cook Time: 5 hours
Total Time: 5 hours 10 minutes
Yield: 4 servings
Serving Size: 4 pieces of chicken

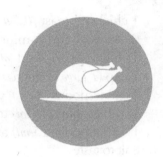

If you've got some cajun seasoning handy (see page 180 for recipe), then use that for this recipe to make it even easier.

INGREDIENTS

- 8 chicken drumsticks and 8 chicken wings
- 4 teaspoons *(20 g)* salt
- 4 teaspoons *(9 g)* paprika
- 1 teaspoon *(2 g)* cayenne pepper
- 2 teaspoons *(5 g)* onion powder
- 2 teaspoons *(3 g)* dried thyme
- 2 teaspoons *(4 g)* white pepper
- 2 teaspoons *(6 g)* garlic powder
- 1 teaspoon *(2 g)* black pepper

INSTRUCTIONS

1. Mix all the spices together in a bowl to make a rub for the chicken. If you don't want your chicken to be spicy, then leave out the cayenne pepper and instead add in more onion powder, but note that the paprika will still make it slightly spicy.
2. Wash the chicken meat in cold water briefly. Place the washed chicken meat into the bowl with the rub, and rub the spices onto the meat thoroughly – try to get it under the chicken skin if you can. The wings and drumsticks work well here because you can rub the spices under the skin easily.
3. Place each piece of chicken covered with the spices into the slow cooker *(no liquid required)*.
4. Set the slow cooker on medium or low heat *(325 F (160 C) if your slow cooker has a temperature controller)*, and cook for 5-6 hours or until the chicken meat falls off the bone.
5. Serve the chicken with the bone on or take the bones out since the meat falls off so easily. Enjoy with some Creamy Cauliflower Mash (see page 145 for recipe).

Nutritional Data (estimates) - per serving:
Calories: 480   Fat: 30 g   Net Carbohydrates: 4 g   Protein: 45 g

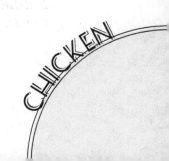

BASIL CHICKEN SAUTE

Prep Time: 10 minutes
Cook Time: 15 minutes
Total Time: 25 minutes
Yield: 2 servings
Serving Size: 1 large plate

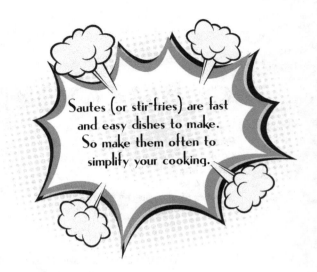

Sautes (or stir-fries) are fast and easy dishes to make. So make them often to simplify your cooking.

INGREDIENTS

- 1 chicken breast *(0.5 lb or 225 g)*, minced or chopped very small
- 2 cloves of garlic, minced
- 1 chili pepper, diced *(optional)*
- 1 cup *(1 large bunch)* basil leaves, finely chopped
- 2 Tablespoons *(30 ml)* water
- 1 Tablespoon *(15 ml)* tamari sauce
- 1 Tablespoon *(15 ml)* avocado or coconut oil to cook in
- Salt to taste

INSTRUCTIONS

1. Add 1 Tablespoon of coconut oil into a large saucepan and add in the minced garlic. When the garlic has started to yellow, add in the diced chili.
2. Then add in the minced chicken.
3. Add in the water and cook until the chicken is cooked.
4. Add to the saucepan the tamari sauce and salt to taste.
5. Lastly, add in the basil leaves and mix it in. Serve with some Cauliflower White "Rice" (see page 143 for recipe).

Nutritional Data (estimates) - per serving:
Calories: 220   Fat: 10 g   Net Carbohydrates: 3 g   Protein: 30 g

CHICKEN PEPPER SAUTE

Prep Time: 5 minutes
Cook Time: 5 minutes
Total Time: 10 minutes
Yield: 2 servings
Serving Size: 1 large plate

INGREDIENTS

- 2 bell peppers, sliced
- 2 cooked and shredded chicken breasts (or equivalent amount of cooked chicken meat)
- 1 Tablespoon *(15 ml)* tamari sauce
- 1 teaspoon *(5 ml)* Chinese chili oil (see page 185 for recipe) (optional)
- 1 Tablespoon *(15 ml)* avocado or coconut oil to cook in
- Salt and pepper to taste

INSTRUCTIONS

1. Add 1 Tablespoon coconut oil into a frying pan on a medium heat.
2. Place the sliced bell peppers into the frying pan.
3. After the bell peppers soften, add in the cooked chicken meat.
4. Add in the tamari sauce, optional chili oil or other seasoning, and salt and pepper to taste.
5. Mix well and stir-fry for a few more minutes. Serve with some Cauliflower White "Rice" (see page 143 for recipe).

Nutritional Data (estimates) - per serving:
Calories: 400   Fat: 13 g   Net Carbohydrates: 8 g   Protein: 55 g

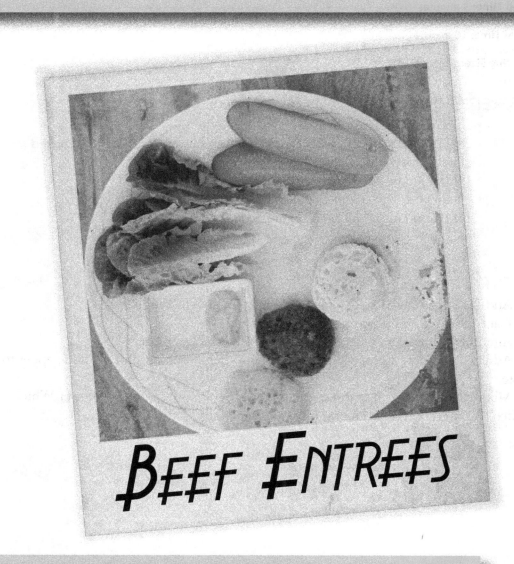

BEEF ENTREES

CHAPTER 3B

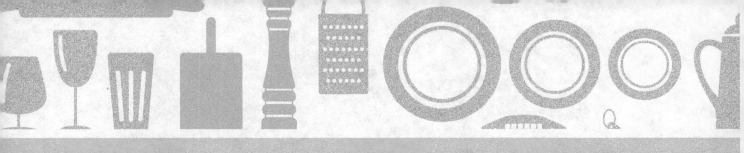

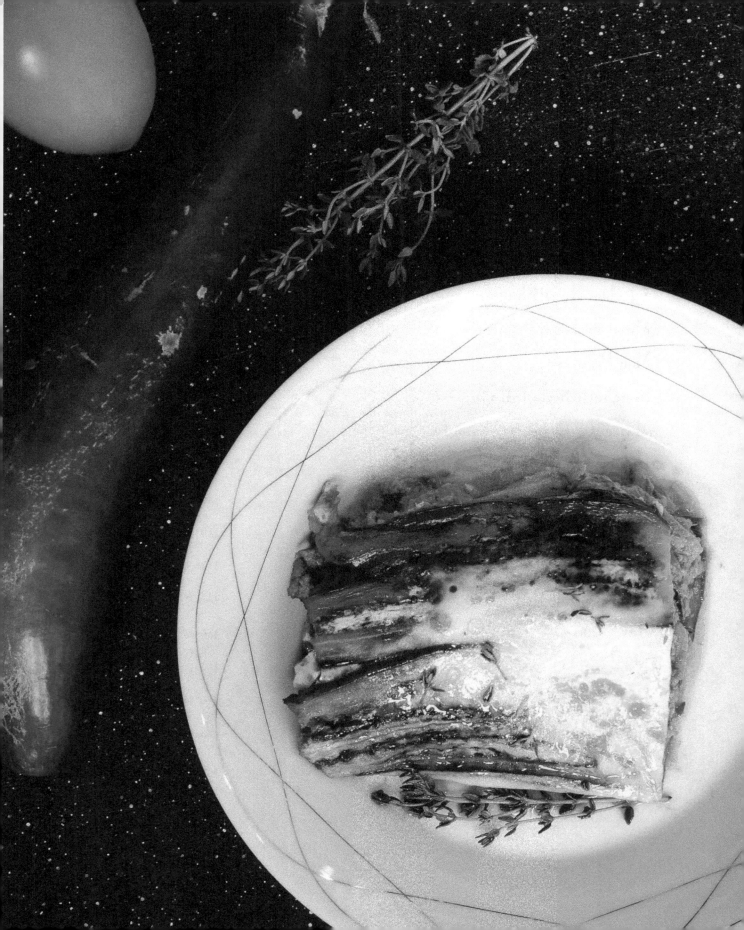

OLD FASHIONED LASAGNA

Prep Time: 15 minutes
Cook Time: 1 hour 50 minutes
Total Time: 2 hours 5 minutes
Yield: 8 servings
Serving Size: 1 large slice

INGREDIENTS

- ¾ lb *(341 g)* ground pork *(or other meat)*
- ¾ lb *(341 g)* ground beef *(or other meat)*
- 1 small onion, finely chopped
- 1 28-ounce *(794 g)* can diced tomatoes
- 2 6-ounce *(170 g)* cans of tomato paste
- 2 Tablespoons *(5 g)* fresh basil, diced
- 6 Tablespoons *(23 g)* fresh parsley, diced
- 1 Tablespoon *(3 g)* fresh oregano, diced
- 1 Tablespoon *(3 g)* fresh thyme, diced
- 1 teaspoon *(2 g)* fennel seeds
- 4 cloves of garlic, minced
- 2 eggs, whisked
- 2 Tablespoons *(30 ml)* coconut oil
- Salt to taste
- 1 large eggplant, sliced into thin slices
- 3 Tablespoons *(45 g)* salt for boiling eggplants

INSTRUCTIONS

1. Place 2 Tablespoons of coconut oil into a large stock pot. Add in the ground meat and the onion. Cook until the meat browns and the onion turns translucent.
2. Then add in the tomatoes, tomato paste, fresh herbs, fennel seeds, and minced garlic.
3. Cook on a low simmer with the lid on for 45 minutes. Stir regularly to make sure nothing sticks to the bottom of the pot.
4. Preheat the oven to 375 F *(190 C)* and boil a pot of water. Add the 3 Tablespoons of salt into the boiling water, then add in the eggplant slices. Boil for 2-3 minutes and then remove and place in cold water *(if your slices are thicker, then you might need to boil for longer - the eggplant should soften so that you can cut it with a fork fairly easily).*
5. Add the whisked eggs into the meat mixture and stir slowly to mix the eggs in. Cook the meat mixture for 10 minutes more and then add salt to taste.
6. Pour half the meat mixture into the bottom of a 13 by 9 inch lasagna pan or a similar baking pan. Top with half the eggplant slices.
7. Then pour the other half of the egg/meat mixture on top of the eggplant slices, and top that egg/meat layer with the rest of the eggplant slices.
8. Cover the tray with aluminum foil and bake for 45-50 minutes.

Nutritional Data (estimates) - per serving:
Calories: 300   Fat: 19 g   Net Carbohydrates: 10 g   Protein: 20 g

the Essential
KETO
Cookbook

BEEF

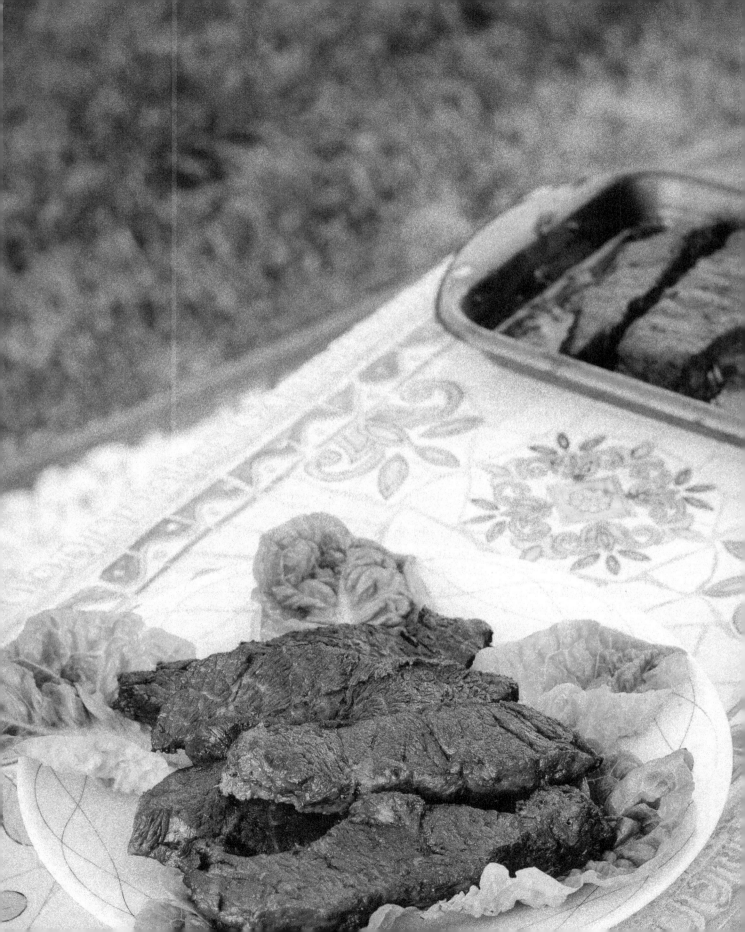

OVEN BRAISED BONELESS SHORT RIBS

Prep Time: 15 minutes
Cook Time: 50 minutes
Total Time: 1 hour 5 minutes
Yield: 4 servings
Serving Size: 1-2 short rib pieces

> Soy sauce can add a lot of flavor to your cooking, but try to use gluten-free tamari sauce or coconut aminos (since they are both gluten-free). While soy is not generally recommended, soy sauce has a fairly insignificant amount of problematic compounds.

INGREDIENTS

- 6-7 boneless beef short ribs
- 1/2 cup *(120 ml)* tamari sauce
- 1/4 large onion, diced
- 2 cloves of garlic, minced
- 2 Tablespoons *(8 g)* parsley, finely chopped
- 1/2 teaspoon *(1 g)* black pepper

INSTRUCTIONS

1. Preheat oven to 375 F *(190 C)*.
2. Place the beef short ribs into a large pot of water and bring to the boil for 5 minutes.
3. In a small bowl, mix together the tamari sauce, diced onions, garlic, parsley, and black pepper. This is the sauce.
4. Place the short ribs onto a small baking tray – pack it as tightly as possible without placing any on top of each other.
5. Pour the sauce over the short ribs in the baking tray so that the short ribs are now sitting in the sauce. The idea is to have 1/2-inch *(1.25 cm)* of sauce at the bottom of the baking tray, which will be cooked off during the baking process.
6. Loosely cover the baking tray with foil and bake for 20 minutes. Turn the boneless short ribs over so the other side gets some of the sauce. Bake for another 20 minutes.
7. Then remove the foil and bake for 10 more minutes until the sauce is mostly gone.
8. Serve immediately or store for use in other dishes.

Nutritional Data (estimates) - per serving:
Calories: 600   Fat: 40 g   Net Carbohydrates: 0 g   Protein: 30 g

the Essential
KETO
COOKBOOK

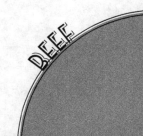

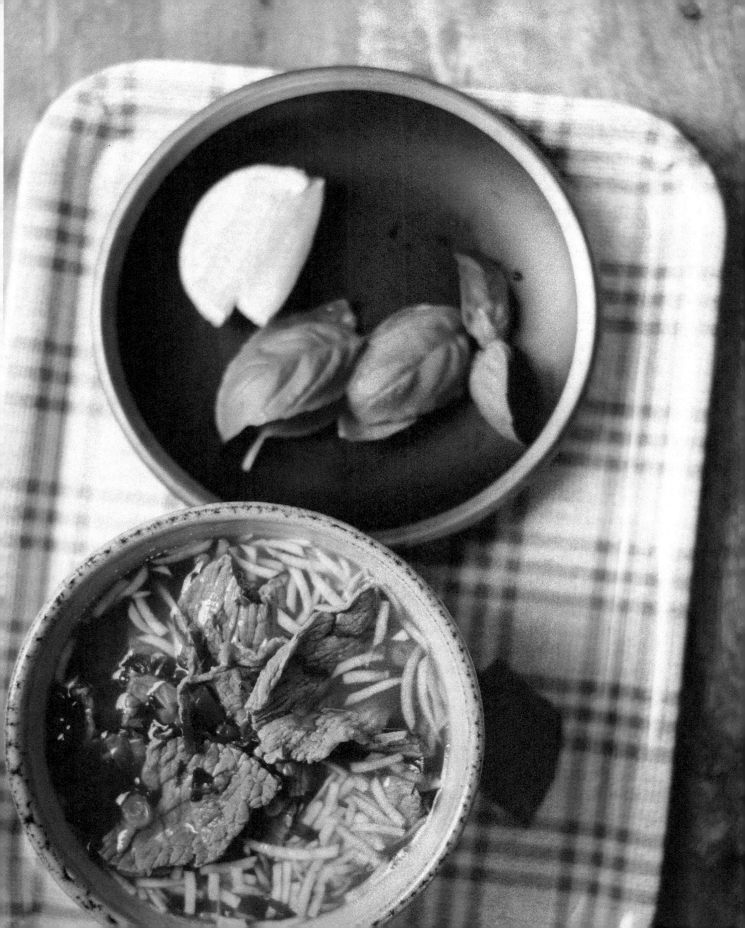

ZUCCHINI BEEF PHO

Prep Time: 15 minutes
Cook Time: 10 minutes
Total Time: 25 minutes
Yield: 2 servings
Serving Size: 1 bowl

INGREDIENTS

- 3 cups *(720 ml)* chicken/beef broth *or* bone broth
- 1/2 lb *(225 g)* beef round, sliced very thin
- 1 teaspoon *(1 g)* fresh ginger, grated
  (or use 1/2 teaspoon *(1 g)* ginger powder)
- 1/2 teaspoon *(1 g)* cinnamon powder
- 2 green onions, diced (scallions)
- 1/4 cup *(8 g)* cilantro, finely diced
- 2 zucchinis, shredded
  (or 2 packs of shirataki noodles)
- Salt and pepper to taste
- 10 basil leaves
- 1/2 lime, cut into 4 wedges

A spiralizer can be a fun way to make noodles using zucchini or cucumber, but if you don't want to splash out for one of those devices, you can use a julienne peeler, a potato peeler, or your food processor's shredding attachment to make your noodle strands.

INSTRUCTIONS

1. Slice the beef round very thinly against the grain (tip: freeze the beef for 20-30 minutes before slicing to get thinner slices).
2. Heat up the broth.
3. When the broth starts boiling, add in the freshly grated ginger, cinnamon powder, and salt and pepper to taste.
4. Add in the beef slices slowly, making sure they don't all clump together.
5. Then add in the zucchini noodles, the green onions, and the cilantro.
6. Cook for 1 minute until the beef slices are done.
7. Serve with the basil leaves and lime wedges.

Nutritional Data (estimates) - per serving:
Calories: 300   Fat: 14 g   Net Carbohydrates: 7 g   Protein: 30 g

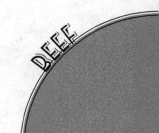

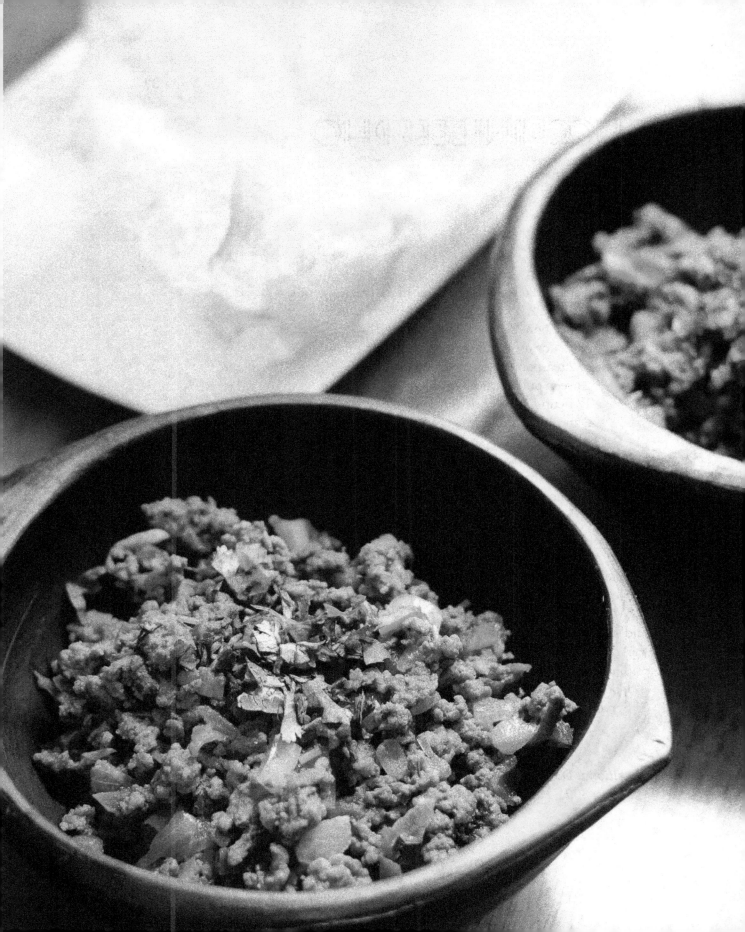

MEXICAN TACOS

Prep Time: 15 minutes
Cook Time: 15 minutes
Total Time: 30 minutes
Yield: 2 servings
Serving Size: 1 bowl

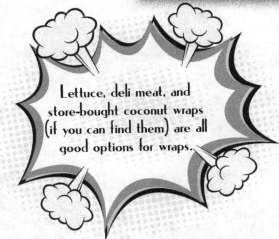

Lettuce, deli meat, and store-bought coconut wraps (if you can find them) are all good options for wraps.

INGREDIENTS

- 1 lb *(454 g)* ground beef
- 1 small onion, diced
- 2 tomatoes, diced
- 1 bell pepper, diced
- 1 jalapeño pepper, deseeded and diced *(optional)*
- 2 cloves of garlic, minced
- 1 Tablespoon *(6 g)* cumin powder
- 1 Tablespoon *(6 g)* paprika
- 1 Tablespoon *(5 g)* dried oregano
- 1/4 teaspoon *(0.5 g)* chili powder *(or to taste)*
- Salt and pepper to taste
- 1/4 cup *(8 g)* cilantro, finely chopped *(for garnish)*
- 1 Tablespoon *(15 ml)* coconut oil to cook with
- Lettuce leaves to serve with

INSTRUCTIONS

1. Sauté the onions in the coconut oil until the onions turn translucent.
2. Add in the ground beef and sauté until the beef is pretty much cooked *(turns light brown)*. Use a spatula to stir the beef to ensure it doesn't clump together. Pour out any excess water/oil produced during cooking.
3. When the beef is pretty much cooked, add in the tomatoes, bell pepper, jalapeño pepper, minced garlic, cumin powder, paprika, oregano, chili powder, salt, and pepper.
4. Cook until the tomatoes and peppers are soft.
5. Garnish with cilantro and serve with lettuce wraps or by themselves.

Nutritional Data (estimates) - per serving:
Calories: 560   Fat: 37 g   Net Carbohydrates: 7 g   Protein: 47 g

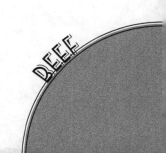

BEEF

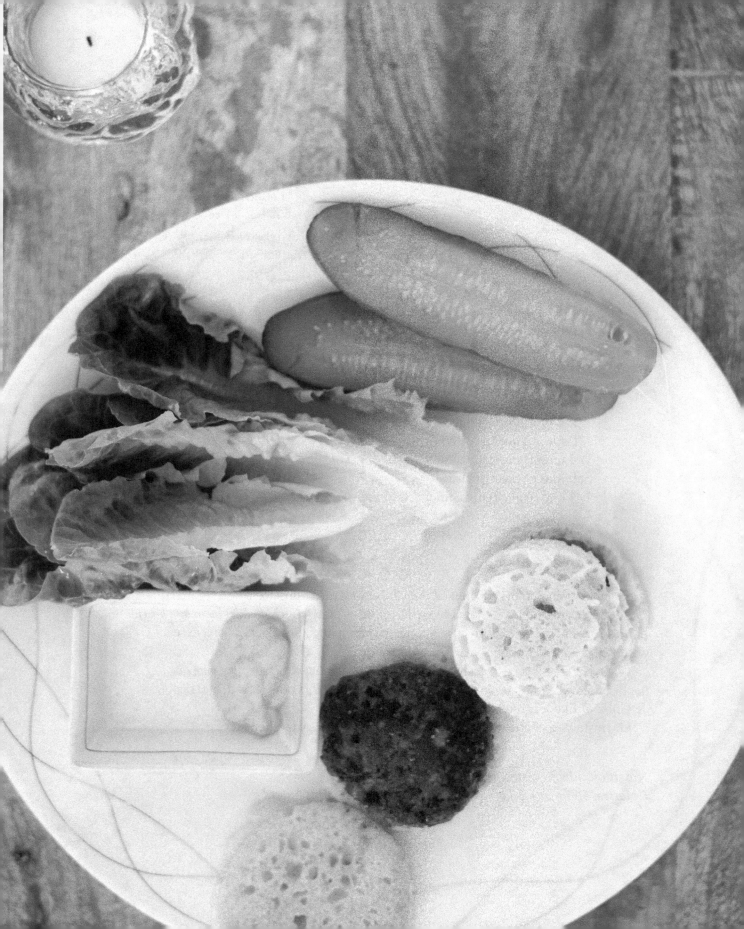

MINI BURGERS

Prep Time: 10 minutes
Cooking Time: 20 minutes
Total Time: 30 minutes
Yield: 2 servings
Serving Size: 2 mini burgers

INGREDIENTS

- 12 oz *(340 g)* ground beef
- 2 Tablespoons *(28 g)* mustard
- Pickles (optional)
- A few lettuce leaves
- Salt to taste
- 2 Tablespoons *(30 ml)* avocado oil *(or coconut oil or ghee to cook with)*

For "burger buns:"
- 2/3 cup *(70 g)* almond flour
- 1 teaspoon *(4 g)* baking powder
- 1 teaspoon *(5 g)* salt
- 2 eggs
- 5 Tablespoons *(75 ml)* coconut oil *(or ghee or olive oil)*, melted

INSTRUCTIONS

1. Make 4 small thin patties with the ground beef (each should be approx. 2-inch across in diameter).

2. Place avocado oil into a frying pan and fry the burger patties on medium to high heat. Fry for 2 minutes on each side until both sides are well browned (this is around medium in terms of rareness for the patties).

3. After the patties are cooked, salt them lightly and place them on a plate to drain.

4. Meanwhile, take 2 mugs and divide the burger bun ingredients between the 2 mugs (i.e., 1/3 cup almond flour, 1/2 teaspoon baking powder, 1/2 teaspoon salt, 1 egg, and 2.5 Tablespoons coconut oil in each mug). Mix well.

5. Microwave each mug for 90 seconds on high. Wait a few minutes before popping them out of the mug. Slice each bread into 4 slices and use as burger buns. (Gently fry them for a few seconds on the frying pan without oil for a toasted taste.)

6. Serve the burgers (2 mini burgers for each person) with the mustard, lettuce leaves, and pickles.

Nutritional Data (estimates) - per serving:
Calories: 850   Fat: 70 g   Net Carbohydrates: 5 g   Protein: 45 g

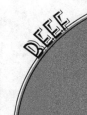

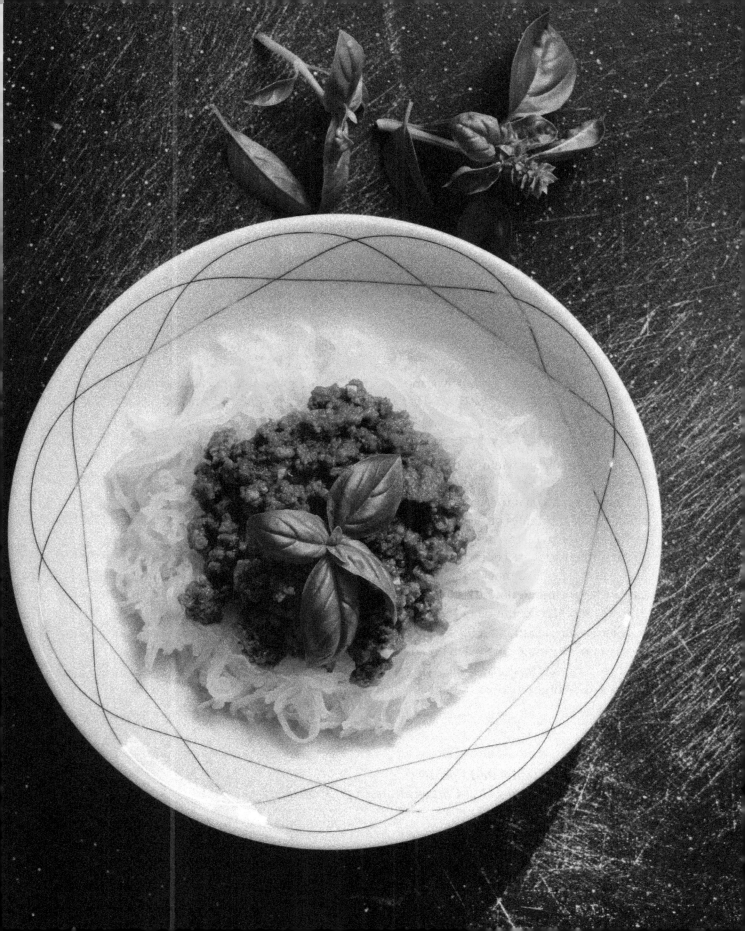

SPAGHETTI SQUASH BOLOGNESE

Prep Time: 10 minutes
Cook Time: 50 minutes
Total Time: 1 hour
Yield: 4 servings
Serving Size: 1 large bowl

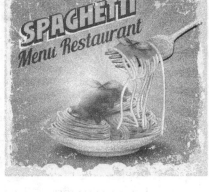

INGREDIENTS

- 1 spaghetti squash
- 2 lb *(908 g)* ground or minced beef
- 1 large onion, diced
- 1 14.5 oz *(410 g)* can of diced tomato
- 1 cup *(40 g)* fresh basil, finely chopped
- 8 cloves of garlic, minced
- Coconut oil to cook with
- Salt and pepper to taste

INSTRUCTIONS

1. Cook the onion in a large pot with coconut oil. Add the ground beef.
2. Once the meat is browned, add the diced tomatoes and simmer with the lid on for 30 minutes (simmer for 1 hour if you have time). Stir regularly to make sure it's not sticking to the bottom of the pot.
3. Meanwhile, chop a spaghetti squash in half, remove the seeds (you can roast the seeds for a snack), cover the insides with a thin layer of coconut oil (you can use your hands to do this), cover with a paper towel to avoid splattering, and microwave each half for 6-7 minutes on high.
4. Use a fork to scratch out the spaghetti squash strands and divide between 4 plates.
5. Add the basil, garlic, salt, and pepper to taste to the meat sauce, cook for 5 more minutes, and top onto the spaghetti squash.

Nutritional Data (estimates) - per serving:
Calories: 450   Fat: 30 g   Net Carbohydrates: 8 g   Protein: 45 g

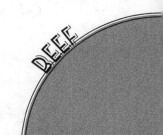

MUSTARD GROUND BEEF SAUTE

Prep Time: 5 minutes
Cook Time: 15 minutes

Total Time: 20 minutes
Yield: 2 servings
Serving Size: 1 bowl

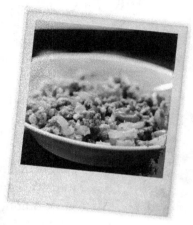

INGREDIENTS

- 0.8 lbs *(360 g)* ground beef
- 5 celery stalks, cut into thin slices
- 10 cherry tomatoes, halved (or 1 tomato, chopped)
- 1 egg
- 1.5 Tablespoons *(20 g)* yellow mustard
- 6 cloves of garlic, minced
- Salt to taste
- 1 Tablespoon *(15 ml)* coconut oil to cook with

INSTRUCTIONS

1. Melt the coconut oil in a large frying pan or saucepan on medium heat and cook the ground beef until all of it turns brown. Stir regularly to get it to cook evenly and to break up any large chunks.

2. Add in the celery slices and cherry tomato halves and cook for 5 minutes while stirring regularly.

3. Break an egg into the pan and stir to mix it into the ground beef mixture.

4. Add in the mustard and garlic, and cook until the pieces of eggs are cooked *(not liquid anymore)*.

5. Add salt to taste.

The mustard makes this recipe amazing! In fact, it's one of my husband's favorites.

Nutritional Data (estimates) - per serving:
Calories: 480   Fat: 30 g   Net Carbohydrates: 6 g   Protein: 40 g

the Essential
KETO

GUACAMOLE BURGER

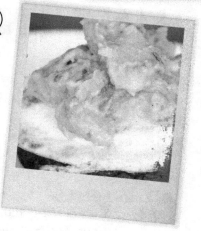

Prep Time: 10 minutes
Cooking Time: 20 minutes
Total Time: 30 minutes
Yield: 4 servings
Serving Size: 1 burger

INGREDIENTS

- 1-1.5 lbs *(454-731 g)* ground beef
- 4 eggs
- Coconut oil to cook with
- 1 cup *(220 g)* guacamole (see page 187 for recipe)

INSTRUCTIONS

1. With your hands, mold the ground beef into 4 patties.
2. Cook the 4 burger patties, either in a skillet with a bit of coconut oil or on a grill.
3. Once the burgers are cooked through, place to the side.
4. Fry the eggs *(preferably in coconut oil)* in a skillet.
5. Place 1 fried egg on top of each burger and then top with guacamole.

Nutritional Data (estimates) - per serving:
Calories: 600   Fat: 45 g   Net Carbohydrates: 4 g   Protein: 45 g

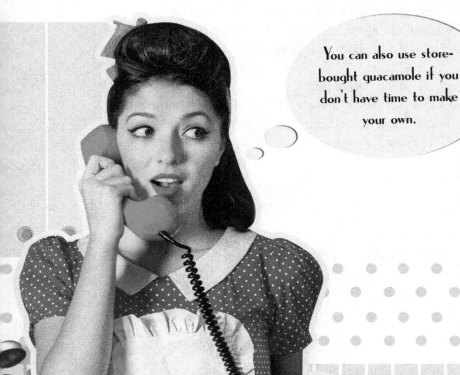

You can also use store-bought guacamole if you don't have time to make your own.

MARINATED GRILLED FLANK STEAK

Prep Time: 8 hours *(for marinating)*
Cook Time: 30 minutes
Total Time: 8 hours 30 minutes
Yield: 6 servings
Serving Size: 8 oz steak

INGREDIENTS

- 3 lbs *(1361 g)* flank steak
- 1 cup *(240 ml)* olive oil
- 2/3 cup *(160 ml)* tamari sauce
- 1/2 cup *(120 ml)* vinegar
- Juice from 1 lemon
- 2 Tablespoons *(28 g)* mustard
- 6 cloves of garlic, minced
- 1 Tablespoon *(5 g)* fresh ginger, grated *(or ginger powder)*
- 1 Tablespoon *(6 g)* paprika
- 1 Tablespoon *(7 g)* onion powder
- 1 Tablespoon *(15 g)* salt
- 2 teaspoons *(3 g)* dried thyme
- 1 teaspoon *(3 g)* chili powder

INSTRUCTIONS

1. Chop the flank steak into manageable pieces if it's not already chopped.
2. Create the marinade by mixing all ingredients *(except the steak)* in a small bowl.
3. Place each piece of steak into a Ziploc bag and divide the marinade equally among the bags.
4. Seal the bags and marinate the steak overnight.
5. When ready, grill each steak by placing on a hot grill or skillet. Try to turn the steaks as little as possible. You can use a meat thermometer to get the steak to the level of rareness you desire. *(We found 3-4 minutes on each side on a hot 500-600 F grill with the lid down worked well.)*

Nutritional Data (estimates) - per serving:
Calories: 700   Fat: 50 g   Net Carbohydrates: 4 g   Protein: 50 g

the Essential
KETO

NO-PASTRY BEEF WELLINGTON

Prep Time: 30 minutes
Cook Time: 30 minutes
Total Time: 60 minutes
Yield: 2 servings
Serving Size: 1/2 of a Beef Wellington

INGREDIENTS

For the duxelles:
- 3 large button mushrooms
- 1 Tablespoon *(10 g)* onions, chopped
- 1 teaspoon *(3 g)* garlic powder
- 1/2 teaspoon *(3 g)* salt
- 2 Tablespoons *(30 ml)* olive oil

Other ingredients:
- 1 9-ounce *(252 g)* filet mignon
- 8 thin slices of prosciutto *(or 4 ham slices)*
- 1 Tablespoon *(14 g)* yellow mustard
- 1/2 Tablespoon *(7 g)* salt
- 2 Tablespoons *(30 ml)* olive oil to cook in

INSTRUCTIONS

1. Preheat oven to 400 F *(200 C)*.
2. Make the duxelles by blending the mushrooms, onions, garlic, salt, and olive oil together until pureed.
3. Then heat the mixture in a pan for 10 minutes on medium heat.
4. Place a large piece of cling-film onto the counter and place the slices of prosciutto side-by-side *(overlapping slightly)* to form a rectangular layer.
5. Spread the duxelles over the prosciutto layer.
6. Sprinkle the 1/2 Tablespoon of salt over the filet mignon.
7. Pan-sear the filet mignon in 2 Tablespoons of olive oil.
8. Spread the 1 Tablespoon of mustard on the seared filet mignon and place in the middle of the prosciutto and duxelles layer.
9. Use the cling-film to wrap the prosciutto around the filet mignon. Then wrap the cling-film around the package to secure it. Use a second piece of cling-film to pull the prosciutto-wrapped package tighter together. Place in fridge for 15 minutes.
10. Remove the cling-film from the refrigerated prosciutto-wrapped beef and place on a greased baking tray.
11. Bake for 20-25 minutes *(it should be pink when you cut into it)*.
12. To serve, carefully cut the Beef Wellington in half.

Nutritional Data (estimates) - per serving:
Calories: 580   Fat: 50 g   Net Carbohydrates: 2 g   Protein: 30 g

the Essential
KETO

BEEF

BEEF BACON STEW

Prep Time: 10 minutes
Cook Time: 2 hour 10 minutes
Total Time: 2 hour 20 minutes
Servings: 4 servings
Yield: 1 large bowl

INGREDIENTS

- 2 lbs *(908 g)* beef stew meat
- 1 carrot, peeled and diced
- 1/4 lb *(112 g)* green beans
- 1/2 lb *(225 g)* celery
- 1/2 pound *(225 g)* bacon, cooked and diced
- 8-12 cups *(1.9-2.8 l)* water or broth (so it covers all the meat and vegetables)
- 3 Tablespoons *(21 g)* unflavored gelatin *(optional)*
- 3 Tablespoons *(18 g)* cumin powder
- 3 Tablespoons *(15 g)* dried onion flakes *(or substitute 1 chopped onion or onion powder)*
- 1 Tablespoon *(6 g)* turmeric
- 1 Tablespoon *(10 g)* garlic powder *(or substitute 3 cloves of garlic, minced)*
- 1 teaspoon *(1 g)* ginger powder *(or substitute 1 freshly teaspoon grated ginger)*
- Salt to taste

INSTRUCTIONS

1. Add the beef, carrots, and green beans to the 8-12 cups (1.9-2.8 l) of water or broth in a large pot and bring to a boil. Then add in the gelatin and the spices and mix well. Place the lid on the pot and let simmer for 1 hour (simmer for 2 hours if you have time). Stir to make sure it doesn't stick to the bottom.
2. When the vegetables are soft, add in the cooked pieces of bacon.
3. Simmer for 5-10 minutes more.

Nutritional Data (estimates) - per serving:
Calories: 800   Fat: 50 g   Net Carbohydrates: 10 g   Protein: 75 g

SLOW COOKER BEEF STEW

Prep Time: 10 minutes
Cook Time: 8 hours
Total Time: 8 hours 10 minutes
Yield: 6 servings
Serving Size: 1 bowl

INGREDIENTS

- 2.5 lbs *(1.1 kg)* beef *(stew meat or short ribs meat)*
- 1 carrot, chopped
- 1 onion, chopped
- 4 celery sticks, chopped
- 2 cloves of garlic, minced
- 1 14.5-ounce *(406 ml)* can of broth *(beef, chicken, or vegetable)*
- 2 teaspoons *(10 g)* salt
- 1/2 teaspoon *(1 g)* black pepper
- 1 teaspoon *(3 g)* garlic powder
- 1 teaspoon *(2 g)* onion powder
- 2 teaspoons *(4 g)* paprika

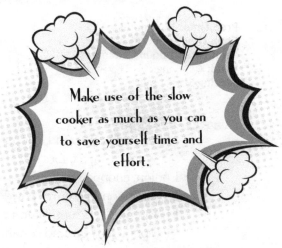

Make use of the slow cooker as much as you can to save yourself time and effort.

INSTRUCTIONS

1. Chop up the beef into 1-inch *(2.5 cm)* cubes if you're not using stew meat.
2. Pour the broth into the bottom of the slow cooker.
3. Place the meat into the slow cooker.
4. Add to the slow cooker the salt, pepper, garlic powder, onion powder, minced garlic, and paprika.
5. Then add the chopped vegetables to the slow cooker.
6. Place the lid on the slow cooker and cook on the low temperature setting for 8 hours.

Nutritional Data (estimates) - per serving:
Calories: 380   Fat: 23 g   Net Carbohydrates: 3 g   Protein: 40 g

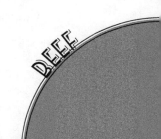

BEEF CURRY

Prep Time: 15 minutes
Cook Time: 1 hour
Total Time: 1 hour 15 minutes
Yield: 4 servings
Serving Size: 1 plate

INGREDIENTS

- 1 lb *(454 g)* beef round, chopped into 1-inch cubes
- 1 onion, chopped
- 1 Tablespoon *(6 g)* curry powder
- 1 teaspoon *(2 g)* ground cumin
- 1 teaspoon *(2 g)* ground coriander
- 1 teaspoon *(2 g)* ground turmeric
- 1 teaspoon *(2 g)* cardamom
- 3/4 cup *(180 ml)* of coconut milk
- 2 carrots, diced
- 1 bell pepper, diced
- 10 button mushrooms, diced (optional)
- 1 Tablespoon *(15 ml)* fish sauce
- 1 teaspoon *(1 g)* fresh ginger, grated
- 2 cloves of garlic, minced
- 1/4 cup *(2 g)* fresh basil leaves, chopped
- Salt to taste
- Coconut oil to cook in

INSTRUCTIONS

1. In a saucepan, saute the beef and onions in 2 Tablespoons of coconut oil on medium heat for 5-6 minutes until the beef is browned.
2. Add the spices, coconut milk, carrots, bell pepper, mushrooms, and fish sauce. Bring to the boil, then cover and simmer for 1 hour until the beef is tender. Add some water if it gets too dry.
3. Add the chopped basil, garlic, ginger, and salt to taste and simmer for 10 more minutes.
4. Serve with some Cauliflower White "Rice" (see page 143 for recipe).

Nutritional Data (estimates) - per serving:
Calories: 440   Fat: 33 g   Net Carbohydrates: 7 g   Protein: 25 g

SLOW COOKER ASIAN POT ROAST

Prep Time: 10 minutes
Cook Time: 8 hours
Total Time: 8 hours 10 minutes
Yield: 4 servings
Serving Size: 1 plate

You can make a large batch of this in advance and use in various stir-fries and sautes.

INGREDIENTS

For the roast:

- 2 lbs *(908 g)* beef round roast
- 1 cup *(240 ml)* tamari sauce
- 1 cup *(240 ml)* beef broth
- 1-2 Tablespoons *(15-30 g)* salt (omit if beef broth is already salted)
- 1 Tablespoon *(7 g)* onion powder
- 1 Tablespoon *(10 g)* garlic powder

- 3-4 star anise
- 10 Szechuan peppercorns

For the sauce:

- 2 Tablespoons *(30 ml)* tamari sauce
- 1 teaspoon *(5 ml)* sesame oil
- 1 clove garlic, minced
- 1/4 teaspoon *(1 ml)* Chinese chili oil (see page 185 for recipe) (optional)

INSTRUCTIONS

1. Put all the roast ingredients into the slow cooker.
2. Fill the slow cooker with enough water to cover the meat (approximately 4 cups, but this will vary depending on the size of your slow cooker).
3. Cook in the slow cooker on low heat for 8 hours.
4. Take the meat out of the slow cooker without the brine and let it cool. Then place into the fridge.
5. Make the sauce by mixing all the sauce ingredients together in a small bowl.
6. To serve, cut the roast into thin slices and lightly drizzle the sauce over the slices.

Nutritional Data (estimates) - per serving:
Calories: 490   Fat: 23 g   Net Carbohydrates: 2 g   Protein: 63 g

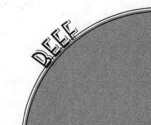

EASY BROCCOLI BEEF STIR-FRY

Prep Time: 10 minutes
Cook Time: 15 minutes
Total Time: 25 minutes
Yield: 2 servings
Serving Size: 1 large plate

INGREDIENTS

- 2 cups *(225 g)* broccoli florets
- 1/2 lb *(225 g)* beef, sliced thin and precooked
  (you can use leftover Slow Cooker Asian Pot Roast (see page 101 for recipe) or Oven Braised Boneless Short Ribs (see page 85 for recipe))
- 3 cloves of garlic, minced
- 1 teaspoon *(1 g)* fresh ginger, grated
- 2 Tablespoons *(30 ml)* tamari sauce or to taste
- Avocado oil to cook in

INSTRUCTIONS

1. Place 2 Tablespoons of avocado oil into a skillet or saucepan on medium heat. Add the broccoli florets into the skillet.
2. When the broccoli softens to the amount you want (I like it soft, but some people like it crunchier), add in the beef slices.
3. Saute for 2 minutes and then add in the garlic, ginger, and tamari sauce.
4. Serve immediately.

Enjoy this Chinese dish with some Cauliflower White "Rice" (see page 143 for recipe)!

Nutritional Data (estimates) - per serving:
Calories: 400   Fat: 28 g   Net Carbohydrates: 6 g   Protein: 28 g

the Essential
KETO

BIFTECK HACHE (FRENCH HAMBURGERS)

Prep Time: 15 minutes
Cook Time: 15 minutes
Total Time: 30 minutes
Yield: 4 servings
Serving Size: 2 burgers

This delicious recipe is based off Julia Child's original bifteck hache recipe published in Mastering the Art of French Cooking Volume 1.

INGREDIENTS

- 2 Tablespoons *(30 ml)* ghee or coconut oil, slightly melted
- 1 onion, finely diced (divided into 2 portions)
- 1.5 lb *(680 g)* ground beef
- 1 egg
- 1 Tablespoon *(2 g)* fresh thyme leaves
- Salt and pepper to taste
- Additional ghee or coconut oil to cook with

For the sauce:
- 1/2 cup *(120 ml)* beef stock
- 2 Tablespoons *(30 ml)* additional ghee
- 1/4 cup *(8 g)* parsley, finely chopped

INSTRUCTIONS

1. Place the 2 Tablespoons of ghee or coconut oil into a frying pan and cook half the diced onions in the pan until they turn translucent.
2. Let the onions cool and then add them (including the oil in the pan) to a mixing bowl with the ground beef, egg, thyme leaves, salt, and pepper.
3. Mix well and form 8 patties from the meat mixture.
4. Cook the patties in a frying pan with additional ghee or coconut oil until both sides are well browned (make flatter patties if you prefer the burgers to be well-done).
5. For the sauce, pour out the remaining oil from the pan, add in the 2 Tablespoons of additional ghee and saute the rest of the diced onions. Then add in the beef stock and reduce the sauce down for a few minutes. Add in the parsley and serve the sauce with the burgers.

Nutritional Data (estimates) - per serving:
Calories: 460   Fat: 36 g   Net Carbohydrates: 1 g   Protein: 35 g

the Essential
KETO

BEEF

CHINESE MEATBALL SOUP

Prep Time: 15 minutes
Cook Time: 15 minutes
Total Time: 30 minutes
Yield: 2 servings
Serving Size: 1 large bowl

INGREDIENTS
- 4 cups (*960 ml*) chicken broth or bone broth (see page 190 for recipe)
- 1 teaspoon *(1 g)* fresh ginger, grated
- 1/2 lb (*225 g*) ground meat of your choice (can also be a mix of different ones - I used 1/4 lb of pork with 1/4 lb of beef)
- 1/4 cup *(8 g)* parsley, chopped
- 5 cloves of garlic, minced
- 2 Tablespoons (*4 g*) fresh thyme (or 2 teaspoons (*3 g*) dried thyme)
- 1 egg, whisked
- 1/2 Tablespoon (*7 g*) salt, or to taste
- 1/4 cup *(8 g)* cilantro, chopped

INSTRUCTIONS
1. Pour the broth into a large pot and set it on a low heat to start simmering. Add in the grated ginger.
2. Meanwhile, in a bowl, mix together the ground meat, parsley, garlic, thyme, whisked egg, and salt.
3. Form approximately 20 meatballs (just a bit smaller than golf-balls) with your hands and carefully place into the large pot of broth.
4. Boil for 10-15 minutes (you can cut one in half to check it's done or use a meat thermometer).
5. Add in the cilantro (and additional salt to taste).

Nutritional Data (estimates) - per serving:
Calories: 300   Fat: 16 g   Net Carbohydrates: 5 g   Protein: 30 g

Pork Entrees

Chapter 3C

PRESSURE COOKER PORK SHOULDER

Prep Time: 10 minutes
Cook Time: 1 hour
Total Time: 1 hour 10 minutes
Yield: 2 servings
Serving Size: 1 plate

INGREDIENTS

- 1 lb (*454 g*) pork shoulder
- 1 onion, diced
- 1 Tablespoon (*5 g*) fresh ginger, grated
- 2 Tablespoons (*30 ml*) apple cider vinegar
- 1 Tablespoon (*15 g*) salt
- 1 teaspoon (*1 g*) black pepper
- 1 cup (*240 ml*) water

INSTRUCTIONS

1. Place all the ingredients into a pressure cooker.
2. Press the Meat/Stew button (normal pressure) and then set the timer for 40 minutes. (The pressure cooker takes a few minutes of prep to get ready and then a few minutes to bring the pressure down, so the total cook time is closer to 1 hour.)

Nutritional Data (estimates) - per serving:
Calories: 550   Fat: 41 g   Net Carbohydrates: 1 g   Protein: 40 g

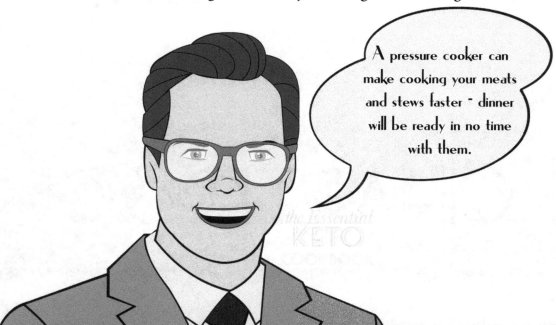

A pressure cooker can make cooking your meats and stews faster - dinner will be ready in no time with them.

PORK AND CASHEW STIR-FRY

Prep Time: 5 minutes
Cook Time: 10 minutes
Total Time: 15 minutes
Yield: 2 servings
Serving Size: 1 plate

INGREDIENTS

- 1/2 lb *(225 g)* pork tenderloin, sliced thin
- 1 egg, whisked
- 1 bell pepper, diced
- 1 green onion, diced
- 1/3 cup *(40 g)* cashews
- 1 Tablespoon *(5 g)* fresh ginger, grated
- 3 cloves of garlic, minced
- 1 teaspoon *(5 ml)* Chinese chili oil (see page 185 for recipe) (optional)
- 1 Tablespoon *(15 ml)* sesame oil (optional)
- 2 Tablespoons *(30 ml)* tamari sauce
- Salt to taste
- Avocado oil to cook with

INSTRUCTIONS

1. Place the avocado oil into a frying pan and cook the whisked egg. Place it aside on a plate.
2. Add additional avocado oil into the frying pan and cook the pork. Then add in the pepper, onion, and cashews. Saute until the pork is fully cooked, then add back in the cooked egg. Then add in the ginger, garlic, chili oil, sesame oil, tamari sauce, and salt to taste.

> You can switch the pork for another meat if you prefer.

Nutritional Data (estimates) - per serving:
Calories: 440   Fat: 31 g   Net Carbohydrates: 8 g   Protein: 32 g

The Essential
KETO

PORK

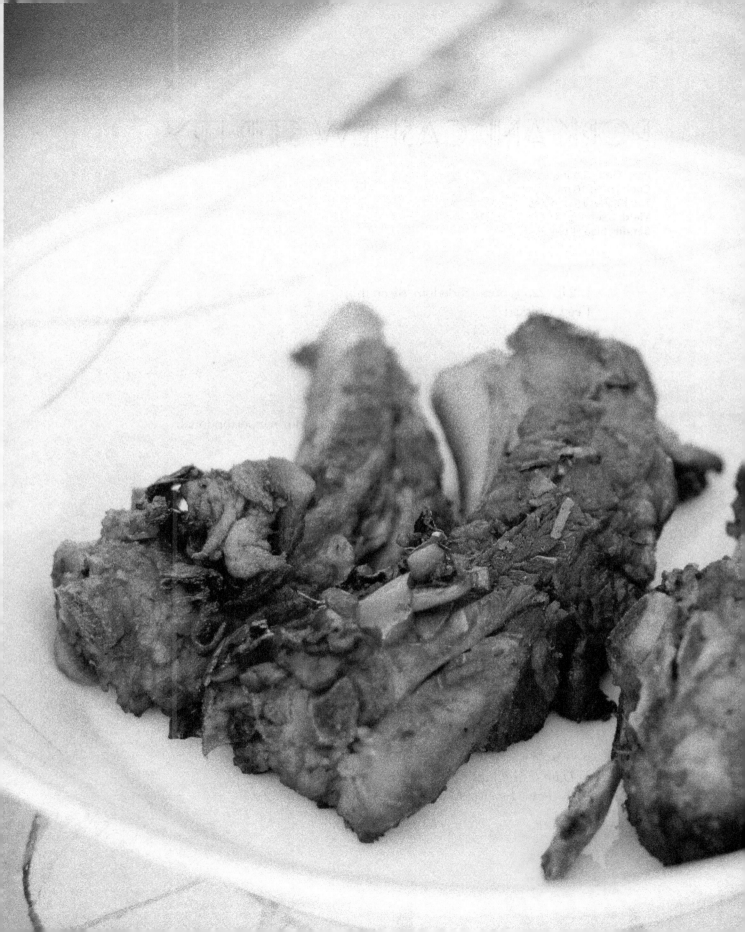

CHINESE PORK SPARE RIBS

Prep Time: 10 minutes
Cook Time: 1 hour 20 minutes
Total Time: 1 hour 30 minutes
Yield: 4 servings
Serving Size: 1 lb (454 g) of ribs

INGREDIENTS

- 4 lb *(1.8 kg)* pork spare ribs *(or back ribs)*, chopped into individual ribs
- 3 star anise
- 20 Szechuan peppercorns
- 2 Tablespoons *(30 g)* salt *(optional)*
- 3 cloves of garlic, minced
- 1/4-inch *(1.25 cm)* chunk of fresh ginger, grated
- 1/4 cup *(17 g)* scallions *(spring onion, diced), divided into 2 parts*
- 4 Tablespoons *(60 ml)* tamari sauce
- 2 Tablespoons *(30 ml)* coconut oil

INSTRUCTIONS

1. Place the ribs in a large stockpot filled with water so that the ribs are covered.
2. After the water starts boiling, skim off any foam that forms on the top of the broth.
3. Add star anise, Szechuan peppercorns, and salt to the pot and simmer until the meat is cooked and soft *(approx. 45 minutes)*.
4. Remove the ribs from the pot but keep the broth (pour it through a sieve to remove all solids). The broth *(by itself)* is wonderful to drink with just a bit of salt, or else you can use it as the base for soups.
5. In a small bowl, mix together the grated ginger, scallions, minced garlic, tamari sauce, and coconut oil.
6. Heat up a skillet *(or wok if you have one)* on high heat and add the ribs in batches to it. Divide the mixture so that you will have enough for each batch of ribs. Coat each batch of ribs on both sides with the mixture. Double the mixture if you prefer more sauce on the ribs.
7. Sauté the ribs on high heat until they brown and no more liquid remains in the skillet.

Nutritional Data (estimates) - per serving:
Calories: 520   Fat: 45 g   Net Carbohydrates: 2 g   Protein: 25 g

the Essential
KETO

PORK

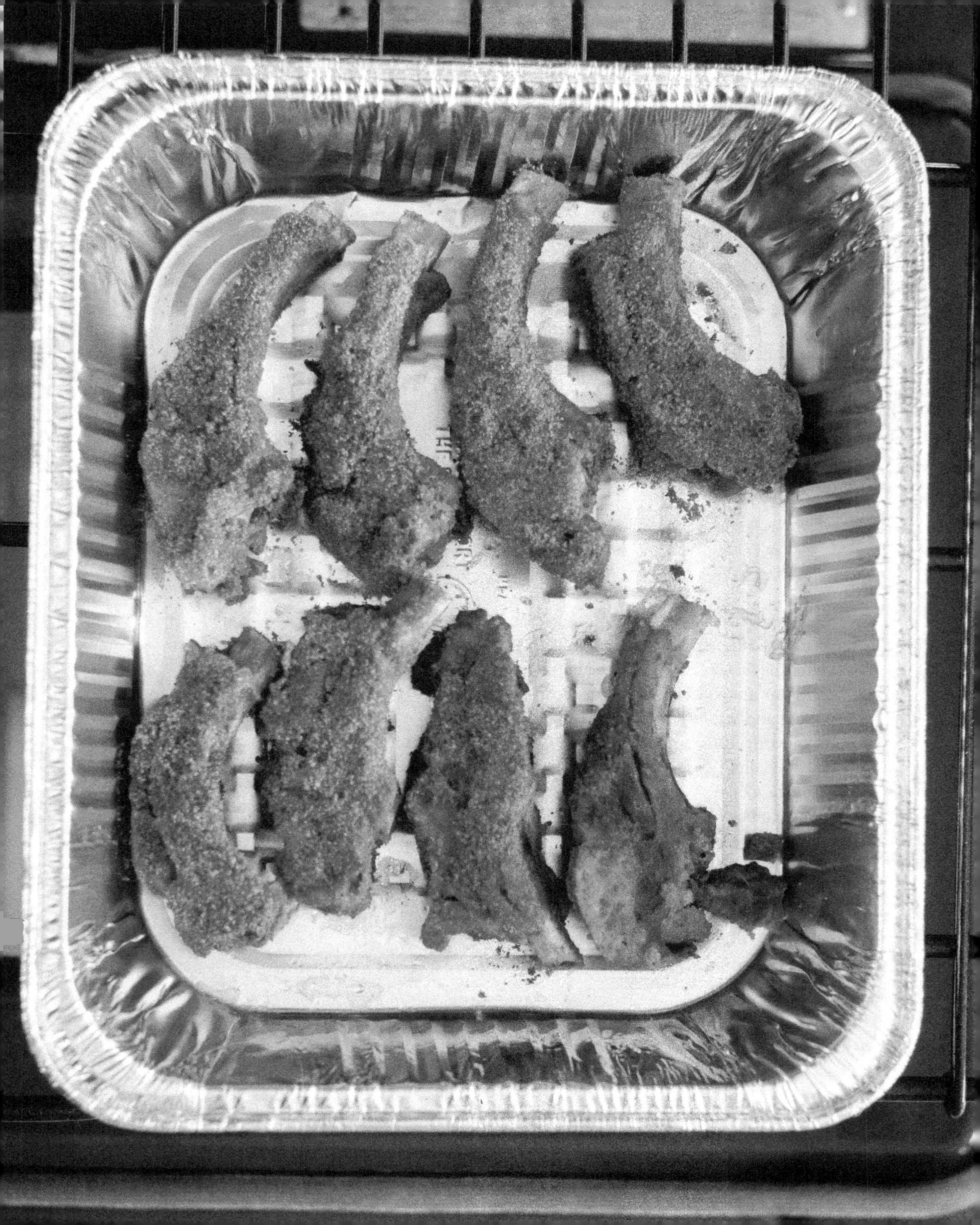

SPICY DRY RUB RIBS

Prep Time: 5 minutes
Cook Time: 2 hours
Total Time: 2 hours 5 minutes
Yield: 2 servings
Serving Size: 1 lb (454 g) of ribs

INGREDIENTS

- 2 lb *(908 g)* pork spare ribs
- 1 Tablespoon *(15 g)* salt
- 2 Tablespoons *(12 g)* paprika
- 1 Tablespoon *(10 g)* garlic powder
- 1 Tablespoon *(7 g)* onion powder
- 1/2 teaspoon *(1 g)* chili powder or cayenne pepper (optional)

You can also use the cajun seasoning (see page 180 for recipe) as the spice rub instead.

INSTRUCTIONS

1. Cut the ribs so that they're in slabs of approx. 4 ribs.

2. Place the ribs in a pot of water (make sure the ribs are submerged in the water) and boil for 1 hour (again, keep the water for broths later). (This is an easy method for cooking tender ribs - there are more complicated methods, but this is the most fool-proof one I've found.)

3. Preheat oven to 325 F *(160 C)*.

4 Mix together the salt, paprika, garlic powder, onion powder, and cayenne pepper to form the rub. Taste the rub to see if you want to add in more of any of the spices.

5. Place the boiled ribs in a baking pan and dip each set of ribs into the rub. Place foil over the baking pan and bake for 40 minutes. Remove the foil and bake for another 20 minutes.

Nutritional Data (estimates) - per serving:
Calories: 520   Fat: 45 g   Net Carbohydrates: 2 g   Protein: 25 g

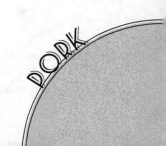

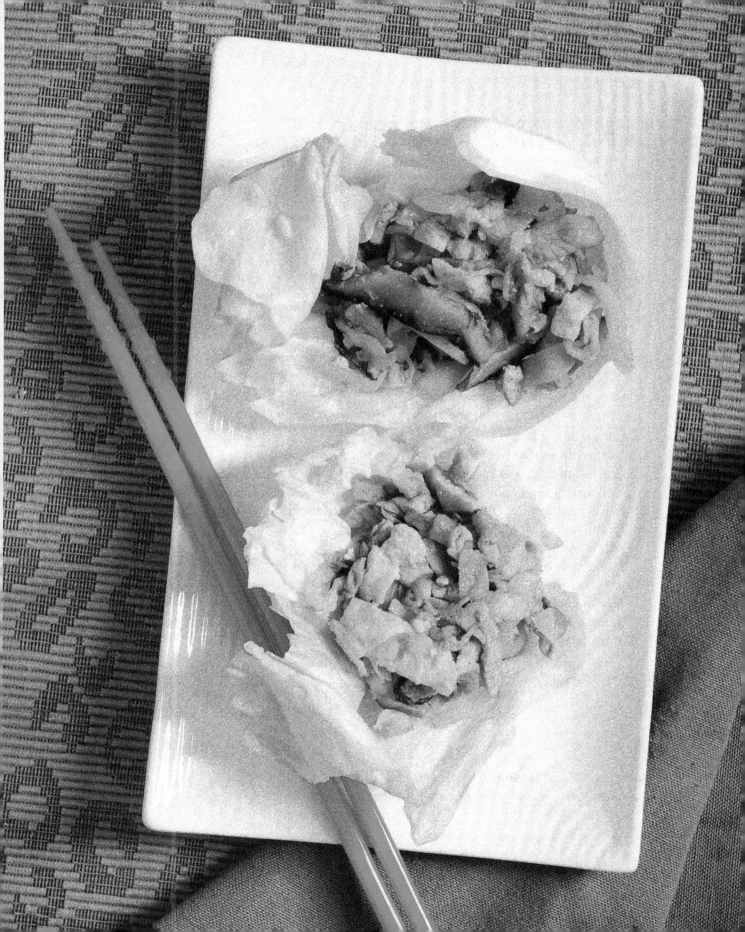

MU SHU PORK

Prep Time: 15 minutes
Cook Time: 15 minutes
Total Time: 30 minutes
Yield: 2 servings
Serving Size: 1 bowl

INGREDIENTS

- 1/2 lb *(225 g)* pork tenderloin, cut into small thin 1-inch long strips
- 3 eggs, whisked
- 15 Napa cabbage leaves, chopped into thin strips
- 1 cup *(89 g)* shiitake mushrooms, sliced
- 1 8-ounce *(227 g)* can of sliced bamboo shoots or asparagus
- 1/2 teaspoon *(1 g)* fresh ginger, grated
- 1 Tablespoon *(15 ml)* tamari sauce
- 1/2 teaspoon *(2.5 ml)* apple cider vinegar
- Salt to taste
- 1 Tablespoon + 1 teaspoon *(18 ml total)* coconut oil to cook in
- 1/4 cup *(17 g)* scallions *(for garnish)*
- Lettuce leaves to serve pork in *(optional)*

INSTRUCTIONS

1. Add 1 Tablespoon *(15 ml)* of coconut oil to a skillet on medium heat.
2. Add a little bit of salt to the whisked eggs and pour the mixture into the skillet. Let it cook undisturbed into a pancake. Flip the egg pancake once it's cooked most of the way through *(it needs to be fairly solid when you flip it)*. Cook for a few more minutes, then place on a cutting board and cut into thin 1-inch long strips.
3. Cook the pork in a teaspoon of coconut oil. Stir with a spatula to make sure the strips don't clump together.
4. Once the pork is cooked, add in the strips of eggs, sliced mushrooms, sliced Napa cabbage, and bamboo shoots. Add in the ginger, tamari sauce, and apple cider vinegar.
5. Cook until the cabbage and mushrooms are soft. Then add salt to taste.
6. Sprinkle the scallions on top for garnish and serve dish in lettuce cups or by itself.

Nutritional Data (estimates) - per serving:
Calories: 340   Fat: 18 g   Net Carbohydrates: 7 g   Protein: 35 g

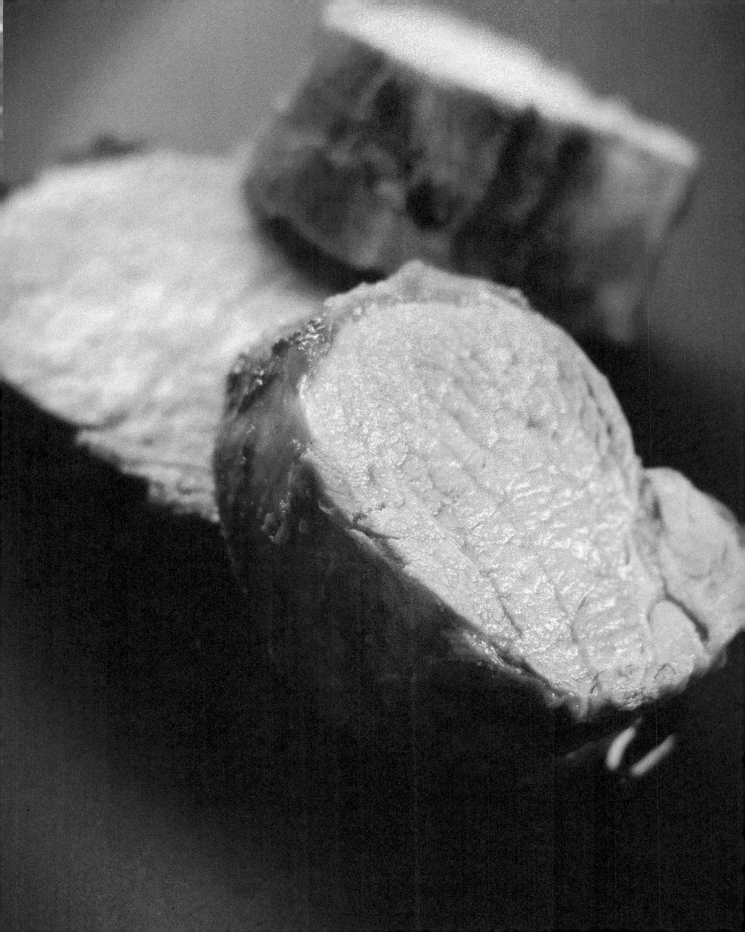

PAN-FRIED PORK TENDERLOIN

Prep Time: 5 minutes
Cook Time: 25minutes
Total Time: 30 minutes
Yield: 2 servings
Serving Size: 1/2 lb pork

INGREDIENTS

- 1 lb *(454 g)* pork tenderloin
- Salt and pepper to taste
- 1 Tablespoon *(15 ml)* coconut oil to cook in

INSTRUCTIONS

1. Cut the 1 lb pork tenderloin in half (to create 2 equal shorter halves).
2. Place the 1 Tablespoon of coconut oil into a frying pan on a medium heat.
3. Place the 2 pork tenderloin pieces into the pan.
4. Leave the pork to cook on its side. Once that side is cooked, turn using tongs to cook the other sides. Keep turning and cooking until the pork looks cooked on all sides.
5. Cook all sides of the pork until the meat thermometer shows an internal temperature of just below 145 F (63 C). The pork will keep on cooking a bit after you take it out of the pan.
6. Let the pork sit for a few minutes and then slice into 1-inch thick slices with a sharp knife.

The pork will be slightly pink on the inside, but if the internal temperature reaches 145 F, then it will be safe to eat (under the new USDA guidelines). The pork will also be tender and delicious!

Nutritional Data (estimates) - per serving:
Calories: 330   Fat: 15 g   Net Carbohydrates: 0 g   Protein: 47 g

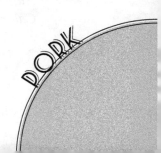

LEMONGRASS PORK RIB SOUP

Prep Time: 10 minutes
Cook Time: 1 hour 30 minutes
Total Time: 1 hour 40 minutes
Yield: 2 servings
Serving Size: 1 large bowl

INGREDIENTS

- 8 cups (*2 l*) water (or use chicken broth)
- 1 lb (*454 g*) baby back pork ribs, chopped into small pieces
- 1 small onion, chopped
- 4 slices of ginger
- 2 1-inch chunks of lemongrass (optional)
- 1 small tomato, sliced
- Juice from 1 lime, or to taste
- 1/4 cup (*8 g*) cilantro, chopped
- Salt to taste

INSTRUCTIONS

1. Place the water/broth into a pot and add in the ribs, onion, ginger, lemongrass, and salt. Place a lid on the pot.
2. Boil for 60 minutes.
3. Add in the sliced tomatoes and continue boiling until ribs are very tender.
4. Squeeze in the lime juice when serving and top with chopped cilantro.

This is an easy version of Thai Tom Saap soup, which is one of my favorite Thai dishes.

Nutritional Data (estimates) - per serving:
Calories: 400   Fat: 32 g   Net Carbohydrates: 4 g   Protein: 23 g

Fish and Seafood Entrees

CHAPTER 3D

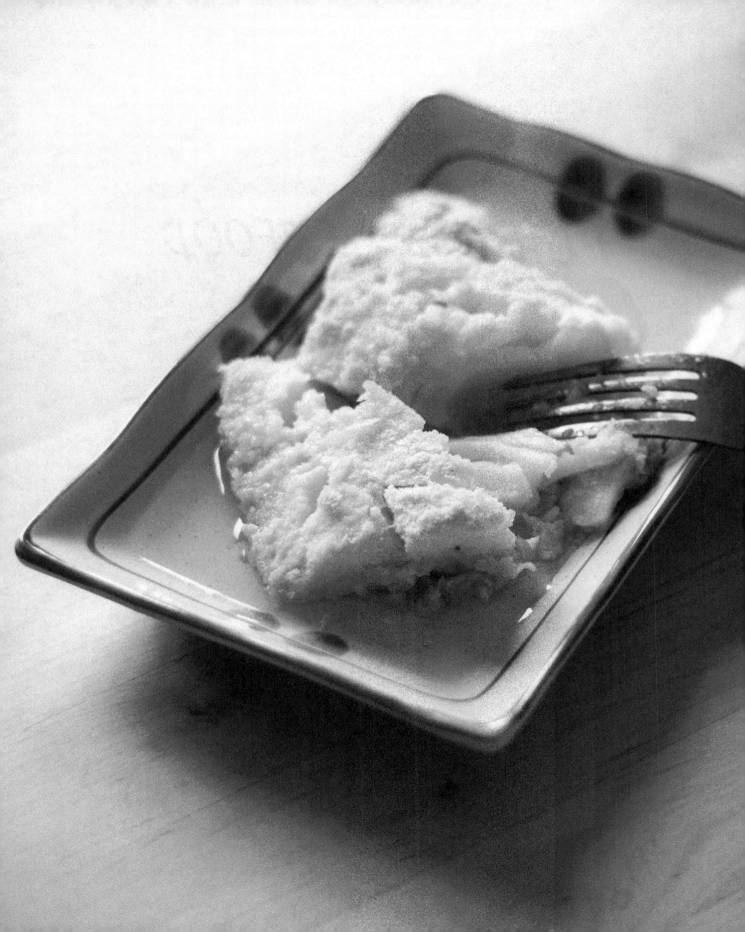

BREADED COD WITH GARLIC GHEE SAUCE

Prep Time: 10 minutes
Cook Time: 20 minutes
Total Time: 30 minutes
Yield: 4 servings
Serving Size: 1 filet

INGREDIENTS

- 4 cod filets *(approx. 0.3 lb or 136 g each)*
- 1/2 cup *(30 g)* coconut flour (or almond flour)
- 2 Tablespoons *(15 g)* coconut flakes
- 3 Tablespoons *(30 g)* garlic powder
- 1 Tablespoon *(7 g)* onion powder
- 1 egg, whisked
- Salt to taste
- 2 Tablespoons *(30 ml)* ghee
- 3 cloves of garlic, minced
- Coconut oil for greasing baking tray

INSTRUCTIONS

1. Preheat oven to 425 F (220 C).
2. In a large bowl, whisk an egg.
3. In a separate large bowl, combine the breading ingredients (coconut flour, coconut flakes, garlic powder, and onion powder). Add in salt and taste the mixture to see how much salt you like.
4. Cover a baking tray with aluminum foil and grease with coconut oil.
5. Dip each cod filet first into the whisked egg and then into the breading mixture and cover it well with the breading. Place the breaded cod onto the baking tray.
6. Bake for 15-20 minutes until the cod flakes easily.
7. While the cod is in the oven, prepare the garlic ghee sauce by melting the ghee slightly and adding in the minced garlic.
8. Pour the garlic ghee sauce on top of the breaded cod and serve.

Nutritional Data (estimates) - per serving:
Calories: 280   Fat: 15 g   Net Carbohydrates: 5 g   Protein: 25 g

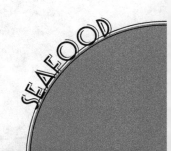

SEAFOOD

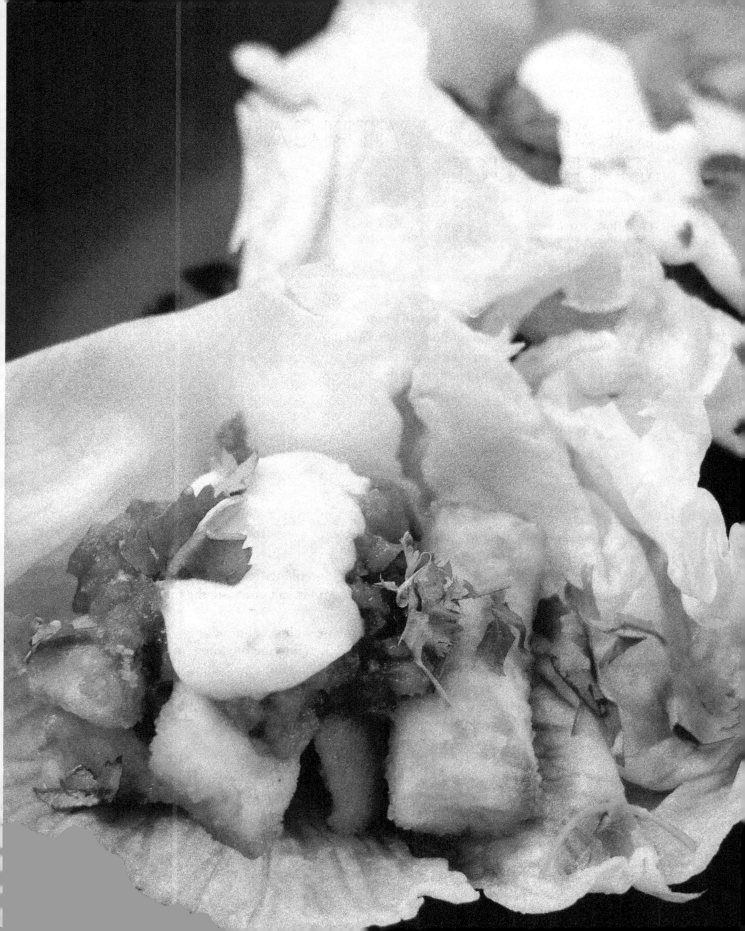

FISH TACOS

Prep Time: 30 minutes
Cook Time: 15 minutes
Total Time: 45 minutes
Yield: 2 servings
Serving Size: 2-3 tacos

INGREDIENTS

For the fish:
- 1 lb *(454 g)* tilapia *(or halibut/cod)*, cut into 1/2 inch by 3/4 inch *(1 cm by 2 cm)* strips
- 1/2 cup *(56 g)* coconut flour
- 1 Tablespoon *(10 g)* garlic powder
- 2 teaspoons *(10 g)* salt
- 2 teaspoons *(5 g)* cumin powder
- Coconut oil for frying

For the white sauce:
- 1/2 cup *(120 g)* mayo (see page 181 for recipe)
- 1 Tablespoon *(15 ml)* lime juice
- 1 teaspoon *(2 g)* dried oregano
- 1/2 teaspoon *(1 g)* cumin powder
- Dash of chili powder

To eat:
- 4-6 lettuce leaves
- 1/4 cup *(60 g)* salsa *(optional)*
- 2 Tablespoons *(4 g)* cilantro, chopped
- 4-6 slices of lime

INSTRUCTIONS

For the white sauce:

1. Mix all ingredients together with a fork.

For the fish:

2. Mix together all dry ingredients *(coconut flour, garlic powder, cumin powder, salt)* in a bowl.

3. Drop the fish strips into the bowl and coat with the coconut flour mixture.

4. Heat up coconut oil in a saucepan on high heat (the coconut oil should be approx. 1/2 inch (1-2 cm) deep).

5. Carefully add the coated fish strips to the hot coconut oil.

6. Fry until the coconut flour coating turns a golden brown color *(takes approx. 5 minutes)*. You should turn the fish strips over after a few minutes since the oil doesn't cover the entire piece of fish.

7. Place the fried fish strips in a bowl lined with a paper towel to soak up the excess oil.

8. To eat, place fish strips on a lettuce leaf with salsa, cilantro, and white sauce.

Nutritional Data (estimates) - per serving:
Calories: 400   Fat: 15 g   Net Carbohydrates: 9 g   Protein: 50 g

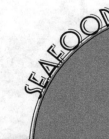

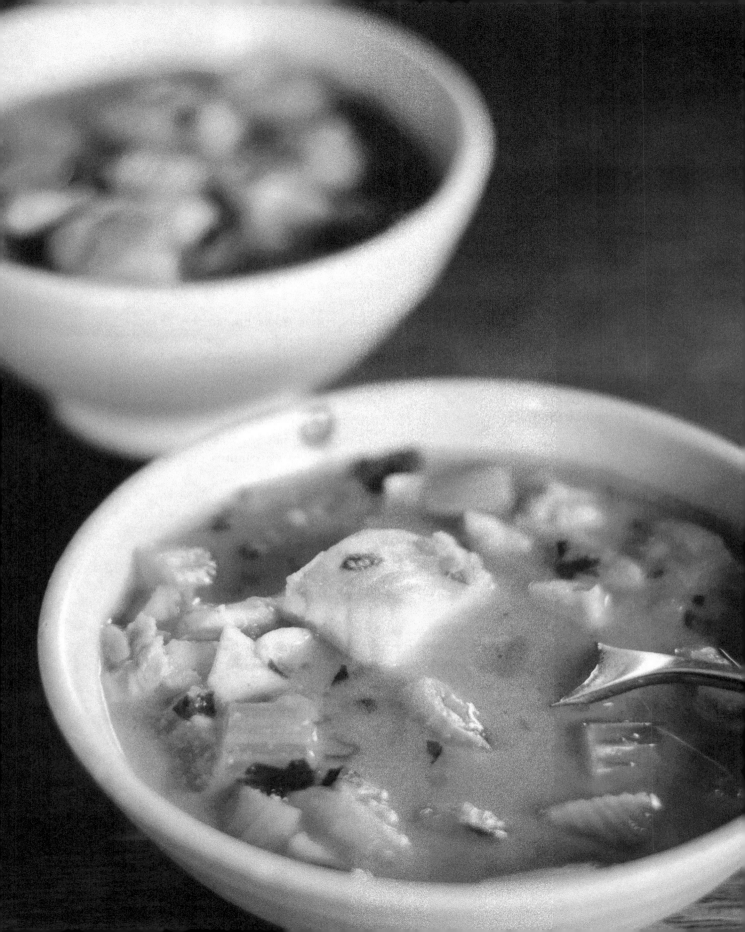

FISH CURRY

Prep Time: 15 minutes
Cook Time: 30 minutes
Total Time: 45 minutes
Yield: 2 servings
Serving Size: 1 large bowl

INGREDIENTS

- 2 cups *(480 ml)* of fish broth (or use chicken broth and add 1/2 teaspoon *(3 ml)* of fish sauce)
- 1 small carrot, peeled and chopped into chunks (optional)
- 3 ribs of celery, chopped into 1/2-inch *(1 cm)* long pieces
- 1 small tomato, diced
- 1 cup *(240 ml)* coconut milk (skim the solid part from a refrigerated can of full fat coconut milk)
- 2 Tablespoons *(12 g)* curry powder or garam masala
- 1 teaspoon *(1 g)* fresh ginger, grated
- 1/4 cup *(8 g)* cilantro, roughly chopped
- 3 cloves of garlic, minced
- Salt to taste
- 1 lb *(454 g)* of tilapia or other fish, cut into large chunks (approx 2/3-inch cubes) (defrost the fish if it's frozen)

INSTRUCTIONS

1. Add the fish broth (or chicken broth with fish sauce) to a pot. Add in the carrot, celery, tomato, coconut milk, and curry powder or garam masala.
2. Bring to a boil and then simmer with the lid on for 20 minutes.
3. Stir in the ginger, cilantro, and garlic. Add salt to taste.
4. Then add in the pieces of fish, making sure they're submerged in the broth. Cook for 5 minutes (the fish should flake easily at that point) and serve. Try not to stir too much as it'll break up the fish pieces.

Nutritional Data (estimates) - per serving:
Calories: 700   Fat: 45 g   Net Carbohydrates: 9 g   Protein: 55 g

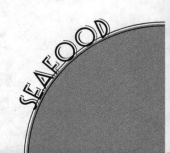

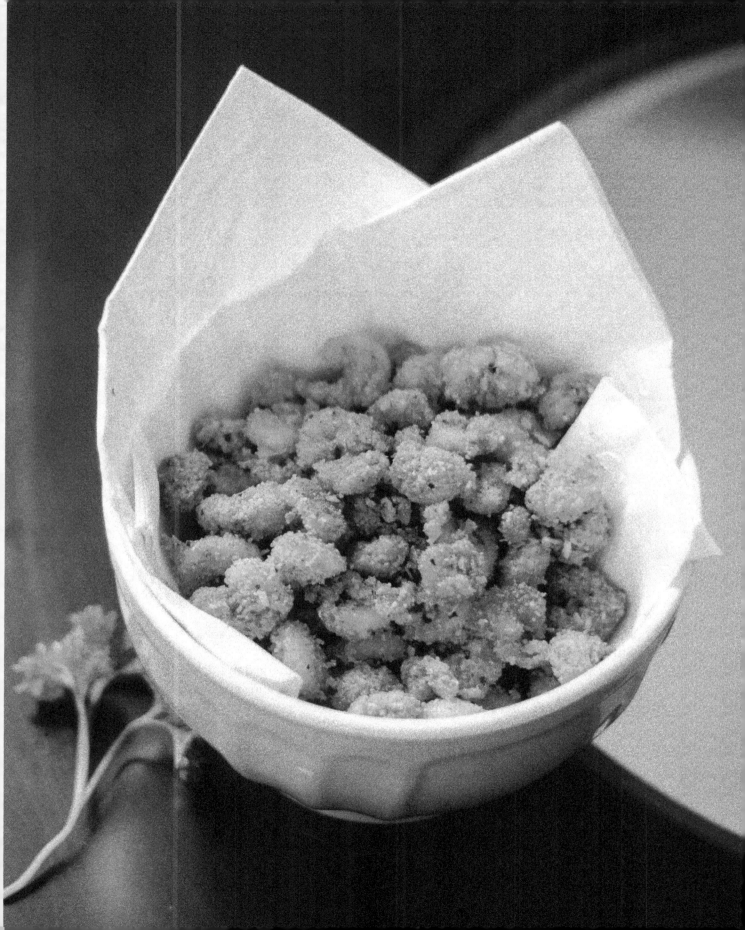

POPCORN SHRIMP

Prep Time: 5 minutes
Cook Time: 20 minutes
Total Time: 25 minutes
Yield: 2 servings
Serving Size: 1/4 lb (113 g) shrimp

INGREDIENTS

- 1/2 lb *(225 g)* small shrimp, peeled
- 2 eggs, whisked
- 6 Tablespoons *(36 g)* cajun seasoning (see page 180 for recipe)
- 6 Tablespoons *(42 g)* coconut flour
- Coconut oil for frying

INSTRUCTIONS

1. Melt the coconut oil in a saucepan (use enough coconut oil so that it's 1/2 inch *(1-2 cm)* deep) or deep fryer.

2. Place the whisked eggs into a large bowl, and in another large bowl, combine the coconut flour and seasoning.

3. Drop a handful of the shrimp into the whisked eggs and stir around so that each shrimp is coated.

4. Then take the shrimp out of the whisked eggs and place into the seasoning bowl. Coat the shrimp with the coconut flour and seasoning mixture.

5. Place the coated shrimp into the hot oil and fry until golden. Try not to stir the pot and don't place too many shrimp into the pot at once *(make sure all the shrimp is touching the oil)*.

6. Using a slotted spoon, remove the shrimp and place on paper towels to absorb the excess oil. Repeat for the rest of the shrimp (change the oil if there are too many solids in it).

7. Cool for 10 minutes *(the outside will get crisp)*.

Nutritional Data (estimates) - per serving:
Calories: 390   Fat: 23 g   Net Carbohydrates: 3 g   Protein: 30 g

the Essential
KETO

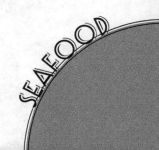

SEAFOOD

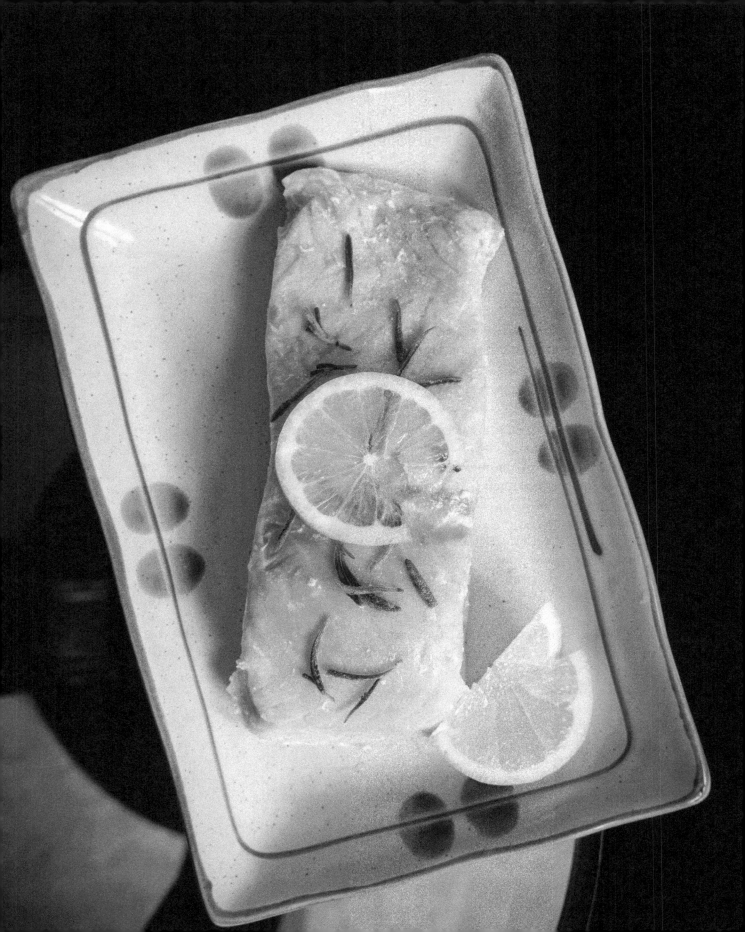

ROSEMARY BAKED SALMON

Prep Time: 5 minutes
Cook Time: 30 minutes
Total Time: 35 minutes
Yield: 2 servings
Serving Size: 1 filet

INGREDIENTS

- 2 salmon filets *(fresh or defrosted)*
- 1 Tablespoon *(2 g)* fresh rosemary leaves
- 1/4 cup *(60 ml)* olive oil
- 1 teaspoon *(5 g)* salt *(optional or to taste)*

INSTRUCTIONS

1. Preheat oven to 350 F *(175 C)*.
2. Mix the olive oil, rosemary, and salt together in a bowl.
3. Place one salmon filet at a time into the mixture and rub the mixture onto the filet.
4. Wrap each filet in a piece of aluminum foil with some of the remaining mixture.
5. Bake for 25-30 minutes.

SUBSTITUTIONS

- Fresh or dried dill can be used instead of the rosemary leaves *(dried rosemary can also be used)*.

This method of cooking salmon keeps it super moist and delicious! You can also easily scale up this recipe.

Nutritional Data (estimates) - per serving:
Calories: 430   Fat: 18 g   Net Carbohydrates: 0 g   Protein: 63 g

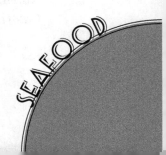

SASHIMI SALAD WITH LIME RADISHES

Prep Time: 15 minutes
Cook Time: 0 minutes
Total Time: 15 minutes
Yield: 2 servings
Serving Size: 1 bowl

Sashimi can be rather hard to find in some places, so use smoked salmon instead.

INGREDIENTS

- 2 handfuls of baby kale leaves (or other salad leaves)
- 1/2 lb *(225 g)* salmon sashimi, sliced into 10-12 slices
- 3 Tablespoons *(45 ml)* tamari sauce
- 2 Tablespoons *(30 ml)* olive oil
- 2 radishes, thinly sliced
- Juice from 1/2 lime

INSTRUCTIONS

1. Place the baby kale leaves on the bottom of a bowl. Top with salmon sashimi and pour the tamari sauce and olive oil over the top.
2. Place the lime juice into a bowl and dip the sliced radishes into it.
3. Place the sliced radishes into the same salad bowl and serve.

SUBSTITUTIONS

- Other salad leaves can be used instead of baby kale leaves.
- Smoked salmon can be used instead of salmon sashimi.

Nutritional Data (estimates) - per serving:
Calories: 290   Fat: 18 g   Net Carbohydrates: 4 g   Protein: 26 g

the Essential
KETO

CILANTRO CELERY SALMON STEW

Prep Time: 10 minutes
Cook Time: 20 minutes
Total Time: 30 minutes
Yield: 2 servings
Serving Size: 1 bowl

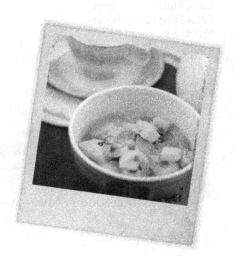

INGREDIENTS

- 4 cups (*1 l*) chicken broth (or bone broth)
- 2 salmon filets (*1/2 lb or 225 g*), diced
- 2 zucchinis, diced
- 4 button mushrooms, diced
- 2 cups (*200 g*) chopped celery
- 1/2 cup (*16 g*) chopped cilantro
- Salt and pepper (to taste)

INSTRUCTIONS

1. Place all the vegetables with the broth into a pot and simmer for 15 minutes.
2. Add the diced salmon and simmer for another 5 minutes.
3. Add salt and pepper to taste and serve.

Stews make easy meals! Throw whatever vegetables you have in the fridge into this one.

Nutritional Data (estimates) - per serving:
Calories: 450   Fat: 12 g   Net Carbohydrates: 7 g   Protein: 70 g

the Essential
KETO

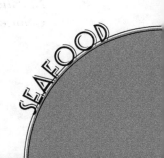

SEAFOOD

FISH AND LEEK SAUTE

Prep Time: 10 minutes
Cook Time: 10 minutes
Total Time: 20 minutes
Yield: 2 servings
Serving Size: 1 plate

INGREDIENTS

- 2 fish filets *(approx. 8 oz or 230 g)*, diced (cod, halibut, or tilapia)
- 1 leek, chopped
- 1 teaspoon *(1 g)* fresh ginger, grated
- 1 Tablespoon *(15 ml)* tamari sauce
- Salt to taste
- 1 Tablespoon *(15 ml)* avocado oil

INSTRUCTIONS

1. Add the avocado oil into a skillet and sauté the chopped leek.
2. When the leeks soften, add the diced fish, grated ginger, tamari sauce, and salt to taste.
3. Saute until the fish isn't translucent anymore and is cooked. Serve immediately.

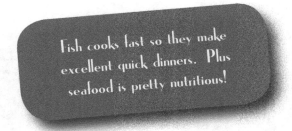

Fish cooks fast so they make excellent quick dinners. Plus seafood is pretty nutritious!

Nutritional Data (estimates) - per serving:
Calories: 190   Fat: 8 g   Net Carbohydrates: 5 g   Protein: 22 g

the Essential
KETO

CUCUMBER GINGER SHRIMP

Prep Time: 5 minutes
Cook Time: 10 minutes
Total Time: 15 minutes
Yield: 1 serving
Serving Size: 1 plate

INGREDIENTS

- 1 large cucumber, peeled and sliced into 1/2-inch round slices
- 10-15 large shrimp/prawns (defrosted if frozen)
- 1 teaspoon *(1 g)* fresh ginger, grated
- Salt to taste
- Coconut oil to cook with

INSTRUCTIONS

1. Place 1 Tablespoon *(15 ml)* of coconut oil into a frying pan on medium heat.
2. Add in the ginger and the cucumber and sauté for 2-3 minutes.
3. Add in the shrimp/prawns and cook until they turn pink and are no longer translucent.
4. Add salt to taste and serve.

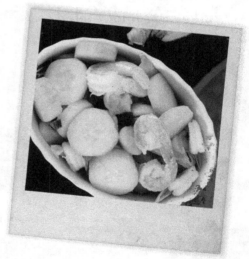

Nutritional Data (estimates) - per serving:
Calories: 250   Fat: 16 g   Net Carbohydrates: 4 g   Protein: 20 g

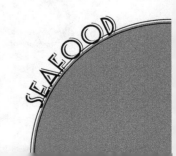

SEAFOOD

OTHER ENTREES

CHAPTER 3E

SLOW COOKER OXTAIL STEW

Prep Time: 10 minutes
Cook Time: 8 hours
Total Time: 8 hours 10 minutes
Yield: 4 servings
Serving Size: 1 plate

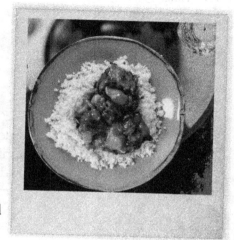

INGREDIENTS

- 2 lb *(908 g)* beef oxtail
- 1 large onion, chopped
- 1 zucchini, chopped
- 1 carrot, chopped
- 2 cups *(480 ml)* chicken broth
- 1 Tablespoon *(5 g)* fresh ginger, chopped
- 5 cloves of garlic, peeled but whole
- Salt to taste

INSTRUCTIONS

1. Place the oxtail, chopped onion, carrot, zucchini, chicken broth, ginger, garlic, and salt into the slow cooker.
2. Cook for 8 hours on the low setting until the meat is tender.

Serve on Cauliflower White "Rice" (see page 143 for recipe).

Nutritional Data (estimates) - per serving:
Calories: 380   Fat: 20 g   Net Carbohydrates: 4 g   Protein: 40 g

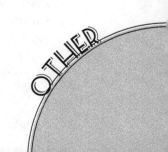

CUMIN CRUSTED LAMB CHOPS

Prep Time: 15 minutes
Cook Time: 15 minutes
Total Time: 30 minutes
Yield: 4 servings
Serving Size: 5 lamb chops

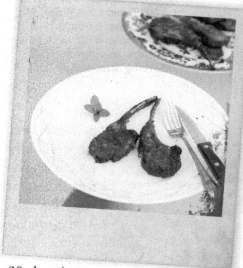

INGREDIENTS

- 2 racks of lamb *(3 lb or 1.3 kg)*
- ¾ cup *(72 g)* cumin powder
- 3 Tablespoons *(18 g)* paprika
- 1 teaspoon *(1 g)* chili powder (more if preferred)
- 1 Tablespoon *(15 g)* salt (less if preferred)

INSTRUCTIONS

1. Cut the racks of lamb into individual lamb chops (approx 20 chops).
2. Combine the cumin powder, paprika, chili powder, and salt.
3. Dip each lamb chop into the mixture.
4. Start the grill and place on the lowest temperature.
5. Place the lamb chops on the grill and cook for 5 minutes with the lid down. Don't let the temperature inside the grill go above 350 F *(175 C)*.
6. Then flip the lamb chops every 2-3 minutes until done to the level you enjoy.

SUBSTITUTION

• Curry powder or Italian seasoning (see page 177 for recipe) can be used instead of cumin/paprika/chili mix.
• The lamb chops can also be cooked in the oven instead at 375 F *(190 C)* for 30 minutes.

Nutritional Data (estimates) - per serving:
Calories: 700   Fat: 60 g   Net Carbohydrates: 2 g   Protein: 45 g

LAMB AND MINT MEATBALLS

Prep Time: 15 minutes
Cook Time: 15 minutes
Total Time: 30 minutes
Yield: 4 servings
Serving Size: 7 meatballs

INGREDIENTS

- 1 lb *(454 g)* lamb meat
- 1 egg
- 1/2 large onion
- 1/2 teaspoon *(1 g)* cumin powder
- 10 fresh mint leaves
- 1 teaspoon *(5 g)* salt
- Avocado oil to cook in

INSTRUCTIONS

1. Place all the ingredients together into the food processor and process well. Form small golf-ball sized meatballs (approx. 25) from the mixture.

2. Place avocado oil into a frying pan and fry the meatballs in batches. Serve with some Easy Bacon Brussels Sprouts (see page 149 for recipe) and with some garlic sauce (see page 178 for recipe).

Nutritional Data (estimates) - per serving:
Calories: 370   Fat: 30 g   Net Carbohydrates: 1 g   Protein: 20 g

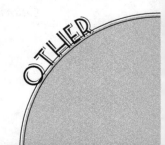

PRESSURE COOKER JAMAICAN OXTAIL STEW

Prep Time: 15 minutes
Cook Time: 50 minutes
Total Time: 1 hour 5 minutes
Yield: 4 servings
Serving Size: 1 large bowl

INGREDIENTS

- 2 lb *(908 g)* oxtail
- 1/2 large onion, chopped
- 2 green onions, chopped
- 6 cloves of garlic, peeled
- 2 Tablespoons *(10 g)* ginger, minced
- 1/4 cup *(60 ml)* tamari sauce
- 1 sprig thyme
- 1 chili pepper
- 1/4 cup *(35 g)* whole almonds
- Salt and pepper to taste
- 2 cups *(480 ml)* water or chicken broth
- 2 Tablespoons *(30 ml)* avocado oil to cook with

INSTRUCTIONS

1. Place the avocado oil into a frying pan and add the chopped onions and oxtail. Cook the onions and oxtail on high heat until the outside of the oxtail starts to brown (approx. 5-10 minutes). Stir regularly.
2. Place the browned oxtail and onions along with all the other ingredients into the pressure cooker.
3. Cook on high pressure for 50 minutes. When ready, follow your pressure cooker's instructions for releasing the pressure safely.

Nutritional Data (estimates) - per serving:
Calories: 470   Fat: 30 g   Net Carbohydrates: 5 g   Protein: 44 g

TURKEY ARUGULA SALAD

Prep Time: 5 minutes
Cook Time: 0 minutes
Total Time: 5 minutes
Yield: 2 servings
Serving Size: 1 large bowl

INGREDIENTS

- 3.5 oz *(100 g)* arugula leaves
- 4 oz *(115 g)* turkey deli meat or turkey breast meat, diced into small pieces
- 10 raspberries (or blueberries)
- 1 cucumber, peeled and diced
- 2 Tablespoons *(30 ml)* olive oil
- Juice from 1/2 a lime

INSTRUCTIONS

1. Toss all the ingredients together in a large bowl and enjoy.

SUBSTITUTION

- This is a really basic salad recipe - you can switch out the meat, the berries, and the salad leaves.

Nutritional Data (estimates) - per serving:
Calories: 260   Fat: 15 g   Net Carbohydrates: 6 g   Protein: 20 g

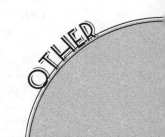

LIVER AND ONIONS

Prep Time: 10 minutes
Cook Time: 20 minutes
Total Time: 30 minutes
Yield: 2 servings
Serving Size: 1 plate

INGREDIENTS

- 1 lb *(454 g)* liver, diced
- 1 large onion, diced
- 2 Tablespoons *(30 ml)* ghee (or coconut oil)
- 2 slices bacon
- Salt and pepper to taste

INSTRUCTIONS

1. Cook the bacon in a pan and then break into small bits.
2. Place the ghee into a frying pan. Add the diced onion and cook until translucent.
3. Then add in the diced liver and saute until cooked. Add in the bacon bits and salt and pepper to taste.

Make this delicious traditional liver and onions dish to get more liver into your diet - it's super nutritious.

Nutritional Data (estimates) - per serving:
Calories: 460   Fat: 24 g   Net Carbohydrates: 8 g   Protein: 45 g

the Essential
KETO

SIDE DISHES

CHAPTER 4

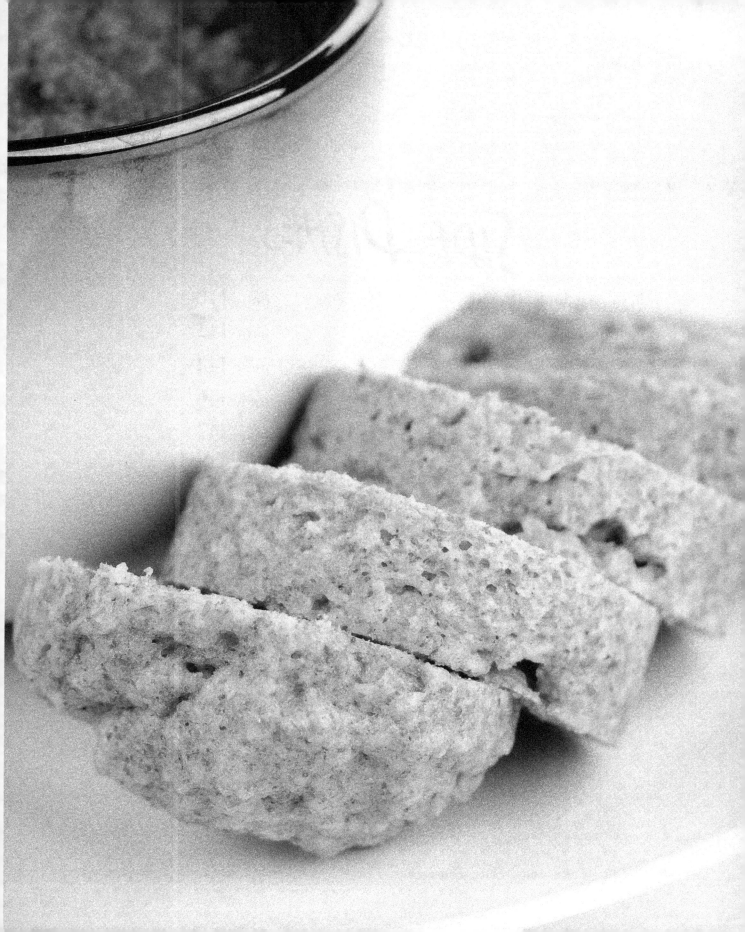

MICROWAVE QUICK BREAD

Prep Time: 3.5 minutes
Cook Time: 1.5 minutes
Total Time: 5 minutes
Yield: 2 servings
Serving Size: 2 small round slices

INGREDIENTS

- 1/3 cup *(35 g)* almond flour
- 1/2 teaspoon *(2 g)* baking powder
- 1/8 teaspoon *(1 g)* salt
- 1 egg, whisked
- 2.5 Tablespoons *(37 ml)* ghee (or coconut oil or olive oil), melted

INSTRUCTIONS

1. Grease a mug.
2. Mix together all the ingredients with a fork.
3. Pour mixture into mug (or mix in the mug to begin with).
4. Microwave for 90 seconds on high. *(You may need to adjust the time for your microwave settings.)*
5. Cool for a few minutes.
6. Pop out of mug gently and slice into 4 thin slices.

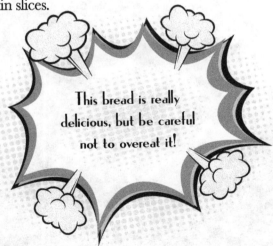

This bread is really delicious, but be careful not to overeat it!

Nutritional Data (estimates) - per serving:
Calories: 260   Fat: 26 g   Net Carbohydrates: 2 g   Protein: 6 g

SIDE DISHES

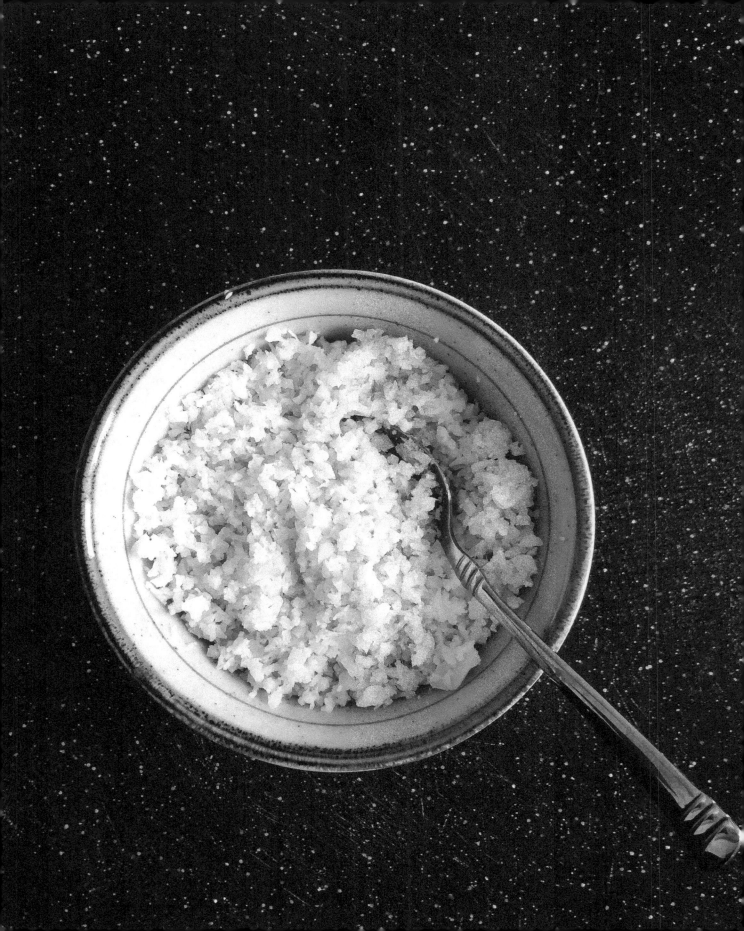

CAULIFLOWER WHITE "RICE"

Prep Time: 10 minutes
Cook Time: 15 minutes
Total Time: 25 minutes
Yield: 2 servings
Serving Size: 1 cup

INGREDIENTS

- 1/2 head *(approx. 220 g)* of cauliflower
- 1 Tablespoon *(15 ml)* coconut oil
- Salt to taste

INSTRUCTIONS

1. Cut up the cauliflower into small florets so that they'll fit into a food processor.
2. Process the cauliflower in the food processor until it forms very small "rice"-like pieces. Squeeze out excess water.
3. Add 1 Tablespoon of coconut oil into a large pot. Add in the cauliflower and let it cook on a medium heat. Stir regularly to make sure it doesn't burn!
4. Cook until tender but not mushy. Add salt and serve.

Pair this cauliflower white "rice" with various sautes and stir-fries.

Nutritional Data (estimates) - per serving:
Calories: 90   Fat: 7 g   Net Carbohydrates: 4 g   Protein: 3 g

the Essential
KETO

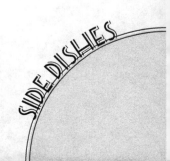

SIDE DISHES

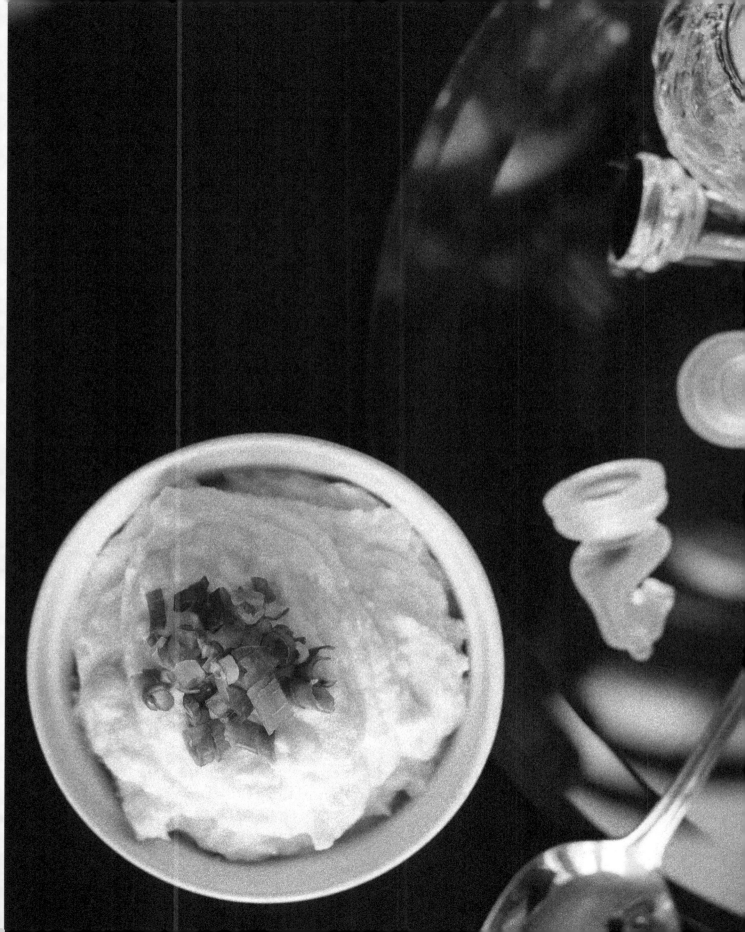

CREAMY CAULIFLOWER MASH

Prep Time: 20 minutes
Cooking Time: 0 minutes
Total Time: 20 minutes
Yield: 2 servings
Serving Size: 1/2 cup

INGREDIENTS

- 1/2 head of cauliflower *(approx. 220 g)*, broken into small florets
- 2 Tablespoons *(30 ml)* ghee (or coconut oil)
- 1/4 cup *(60 ml)* coconut milk
    (from a can shaken and at room temperature)
- 1/4 teaspoon *(1 ml)* vanilla extract
- Chives or scallions (chopped spring onion), finely chopped (optional)
- Salt to taste

INSTRUCTIONS

1. Place the cauliflower florets into a large microwaveable bowl with 1/4 cup of water at the bottom. Microwave on high until they are softened (around 10-12 minutes). Check every 3 minutes to make sure there's water in the bowl still. Alternatively, you can steam the cauliflower florets in a steamer.

2. Place the softened cauliflower along with the melted ghee, coconut milk, vanilla extract, and salt into a blender and blend until smooth.

3. Top with chives or scallions.

This cauliflower mash is super creamy and delicious - in fact, most people don't even realize it's made from cauliflower!

Nutritional Data (estimates) - per serving:
Calories: 200   Fat: 20 g   Net Carbohydrates: 4 g   Protein: 4 g

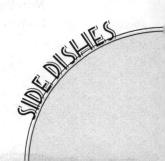
SIDE DISHES

SPINACH ALMOND SAUTE

Prep Time: 0 minutes
Cook Time: 10 minutes
Total Time: 10 minutes
Yield: 2 servings
Serving Size: 1 cup

INGREDIENTS

- 1 lb *(454 g)* spinach leaves
- 3 Tablespoons *(12 g)* almond slices
- Salt to taste
- 1 Tablespoon *(15 ml)* avocado oil for cooking

INSTRUCTIONS

1. Place the 1 Tablespoon of avocado oil into a large pot on medium heat.
2. Add in the spinach and let it cook down.
3. Once the spinach is cooked down, add the salt to taste and stir.
4. Before serving, stir in the almond slices.

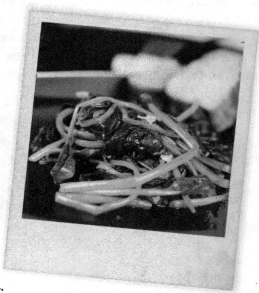

Nutritional Data (estimates) - per serving:
Calories: 150   Fat: 11 g   Net Carbohydrates: 4 g   Protein: 8 g

LEMON ASPARAGUS SAUTE WITH BACON

Prep Time: 5 minutes
Cook Time: 15 minutes
Total Time: 20 minutes
Yield: 4 servings
Serving Size: 1 cup

INGREDIENTS

- 20 stalks of asparagus (approx.), chop off the end of the stalks and chop into small chunks
- 1 lemon
- 1/2 cup *(50 g)* bacon bits/pieces, precooked
- Salt to taste
- Olive oil or bacon fat to cook with

INSTRUCTIONS

1. Saute the asparagus in approx. 2 Tablespoons of olive oil.
2. When the asparagus slices are tender, squeeze in the juice from 1 lemon (taste after squeezing in 1/2 a lemon to make sure how much more lemon juice you want).
3. Add in the bacon bits and saute for 2-3 minutes more.
4. Add salt to taste.

You can use leftover meats instead of bacon for this dish.

Nutritional Data (estimates) - per serving:
Calories: 200   Fat: 15 g   Net Carbohydrates: 3 g   Protein: 13 g

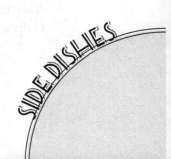

GARLIC LEMON BROCCOLINI SAUTE

Prep Time: 5 minutes
Cook Time: 10 minutes
Total Time: 15 minutes
Yield: 2 servings
Serving Size: 1 plate

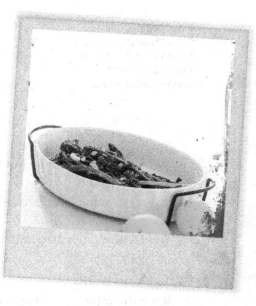

INGREDIENTS

- 1/2 lb *(225 g)* broccolini
- 3 cloves of garlic, minced
- 1 Tablespoon *(15 ml)* lemon juice
- 1 Tablespoon *(10 g)* garlic powder (optional)
- 2 Tablespoons *(30 ml)* olive oil
- Salt and pepper to taste

INSTRUCTIONS

1. Add the olive oil into the skillet on medium heat.
2. Add in the broccolini and saute for 5 minutes (parboil the broccolini first if you prefer it softer).
3. Add in the minced garlic, lemon juice, garlic powder, salt, and pepper.
4. Saute for a few more minutes and serve immediately.

SUBSTITUTIONS

- Chopped broccoli can be used instead of broccolini.

Nutritional Data (estimates) - per serving:
Calories: 150   Fat: 10 g   Net Carbohydrates: 6 g   Protein: 5 g

EASY BACON BRUSSELS SPROUTS

Prep Time: 5 minutes
Cook Time: 20 minutes
Total Time: 25 minutes
Yield: 6 servings
Serving Size: 1 cup *(approx.)*

INGREDIENTS

- 2 lbs *(908 g)* Brussels sprouts
- 1 lb *(454 g)* bacon, uncooked

INSTRUCTIONS

1. Boil the Brussels sprouts for 10 minutes until tender.

2. While the Brussels sprouts are boiling, chop the bacon into small pieces *(approx. 1/2-inch wide)*, and cook the bacon pieces in a large pot on medium heat. When the bacon is crispy, add in the drained Brussels sprouts.

3. Cook for 10 more minutes on high heat, stirring occasionally to make sure nothing gets burnt on the bottom of the pan.

This is one of my favorite recipes - it's easy to make and absolutely delicious. Plus, you can make a large batch of it and refrigerate it to eat over several days.

Nutritional Data (estimates) - per serving:
Calories: 400   Fat: 35 g   Net Carbohydrates: 6 g   Protein: 14 g

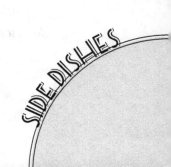

REFRESHING CUCUMBER SALAD

Prep Time: 10 minutes
Cooking Time: 0 minutes
Total Time: 10 minutes
Yield: 6 servings
Serving Size: 1 cup

INGREDIENTS

- 3 small cucumbers *(or 2 large cucumbers)*, peeled
- 12 cloves of garlic, minced
- 1 teaspoon *(5 g)* salt
- 3 Tablespoons *(45 ml)* olive oil

INSTRUCTIONS

1. Cube the cucumbers.
2. Mix the cucumbers, minced garlic, salt, and olive oil together.
3. Best served chilled.

SUBSTITUTIONS

- Sesame oil can be used instead of olive oil.

Nutritional Data (estimates) - per serving:
Calories: 80   Fat: 7 g   Net Carbohydrates: 2 g   Protein: 0 g

the Essential
KETO

GARLIC ZUCCHINI SAUTE

Prep Time: 5 minutes
Cook Time: 12 minutes
Total Time: 17 minutes
Yield: 4 servings
Serving Size: 1-2 cups

INGREDIENTS

- 2 lb *(908 g)* zucchini, chopped into small pieces or slices
- 6 cloves of garlic, minced
- Olive oil to saute in

INSTRUCTIONS

1. Pour 3-4 tablespoons of olive oil into a skillet on medium to high heat.
2. Place the baby squash/zucchini pieces into the skillet and saute until they soften (approx. 10 minutes).
3. Add the garlic and saute for 1-2 minutes more.

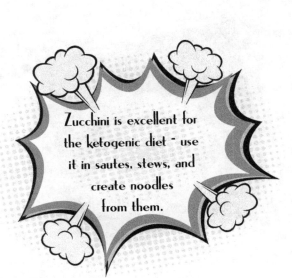

Zucchini is excellent for the ketogenic diet - use it in sautes, stews, and create noodles from them.

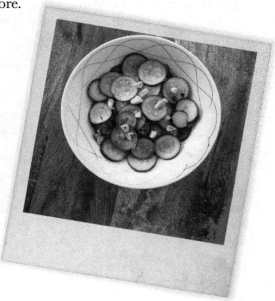

Nutritional Data (estimates) - per serving:
Calories: 70   Fat: 4 g   Net Carbohydrates: 4 g   Protein: 0 g

the Essential
KETO

SIDE DISHES

EASY EGG SALAD

Prep Time: 5 minutes
Cook Time: 20 minutes
Total Time: 25 minutes
Yield: 2 servings
Serving Size: 2 eggs worth

INGREDIENTS

- 4 hard boiled eggs, peeled
- 1/2 Tablespoon *(7 g)* mustard (add more to taste)
- 1/2 Tablespoon *(7 ml)* mayo (see page 181 for recipe)
- 1 Tablespoon pickles, chopped (optional)
- Dash of smoked paprika (optional)
- Salt and pepper to taste

INSTRUCTIONS

1. Cut up the hard boiled eggs into small pieces.
2. In a bowl, combine with the mustard, mayo, pickles, and seasoning. Mix well.

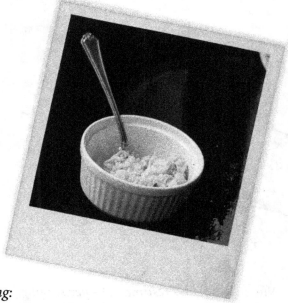

Nutritional Data (estimates) - per serving:
Calories: 160   Fat: 11 g   Net Carbohydrates: 1 g   Protein: 13 g

ROASTED TURMERIC CAULIFLOWER

Prep Time: 15 minutes
Cook Time: 1 hour 15 minutes
Total Time: 1 hour 30 minutes
Servings: 4 servings
Yield: 1 small bowl

> Turmeric goes really well with cauliflower. In fact, you can add turmeric to your cauliflower mash (see page 144 for recipe) as well.

INGREDIENTS

- Half of a large cauliflower *(approx. 220 g)*
- 2 teaspoons *(4 g)* turmeric
- 2 teaspoons *(10 g)* salt
- 2 Tablespoons *(30 ml)* olive oil

INSTRUCTIONS

1. Preheat oven to 350 F *(175 C)*.
2. Separate the cauliflower florets from the cauliflower stem. Discard the stem.
3. Combine the cauliflower florets with the turmeric, salt, and olive oil.
4. Place in baking dish *(spread out the cauliflower so they're not on top of each other)*.
5. Cover the baking dish with foil.
6. Bake for 75 minutes.

Nutritional Data (estimates) - per serving:
Calories: 90   Fat: 7 g   Net Carbohydrates: 3 g   Protein: 0 g

SIDE DISHES

QUICK STEWED NAPA CABBAGE

Prep Time: 10 minutes
Cook Time: 20 minutes
Total Time: 30 minutes
Yield: 4 servings
Serving Size: 1 cup

INGREDIENTS

- 1 head of Napa cabbage (also known as Chinese cabbage), chop off the bottom end and then chop roughly into 1-inch *(2.5 cm)* chunks (or use regular white cabbage)
- 1 small tomato, diced
- 1 bell pepper, diced
- 3 Tablespoons *(45 ml)* chicken broth (optional)
- Salt and pepper to taste
- Coconut oil to cook with

INSTRUCTIONS

1. Add 2 Tablespoons of coconut oil to a large pot.
2. Add in the cabbage, tomato, and bell pepper, and cook on a medium-high heat. The cabbage will release a lot of water and will decrease in size.
3. Add in the chicken broth after 10 minutes (optional).
4. Cook for around 20 minutes until the cabbage is very soft and some of the water has evaporated.
5. Add in salt and pepper to taste.
6. Serve with a little bit of the broth.

Nutritional Data (estimates) - per serving:
Calories: 70   Fat: 4 g   Net Carbohydrates: 6 g   Protein: 3 g

SUPER FAST AVOCADO SALAD

Prep Time: 5 minutes
Cooking Time: 0 minutes
Total Time: 5 minutes
Yield: 2 servings
Serving Size: 1 cup

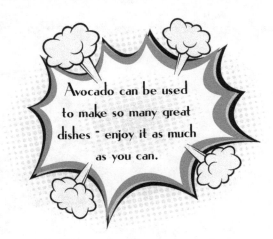

Avocado can be used to make so many great dishes - enjoy it as much as you can.

INGREDIENTS

- 1 ripe avocado
- 1 Tablespoon *(15 ml)* olive oil
- 1/2 Tablespoon *(7 ml)* lemon juice
- Salt to taste

INSTRUCTIONS

1. Cut a ripe avocado in half.
2. Remove the pit, and using a small knife carefully score each half into cubes. Then use a spoon to scoop out the avocado cubes.
3. Toss the avocado cubes with olive oil, balsamic vinegar, and salt.

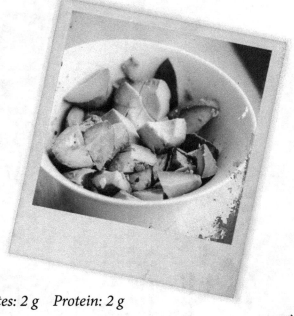

Nutritional Data (estimates) - per serving:
Calories: 220   Fat: 21 g   Net Carbohydrates: 2 g   Protein: 2 g

the Essential
KETO
COOKBOOK

SIDE DISHES

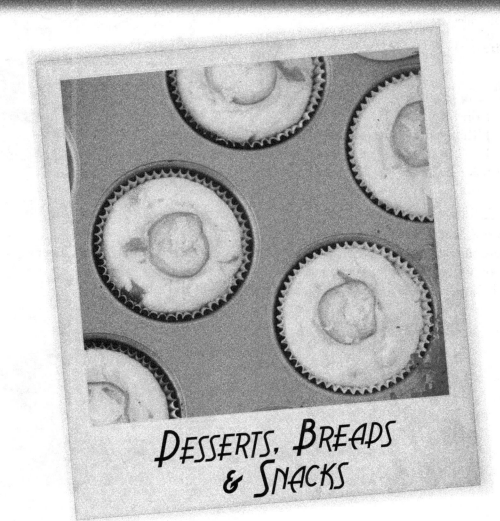

DESSERTS, BREADS
& SNACKS

CHAPTER 5

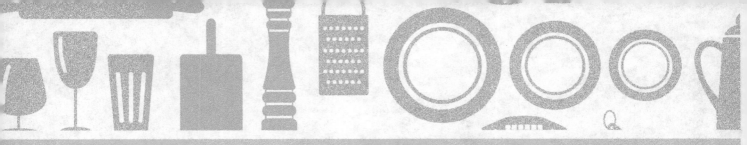

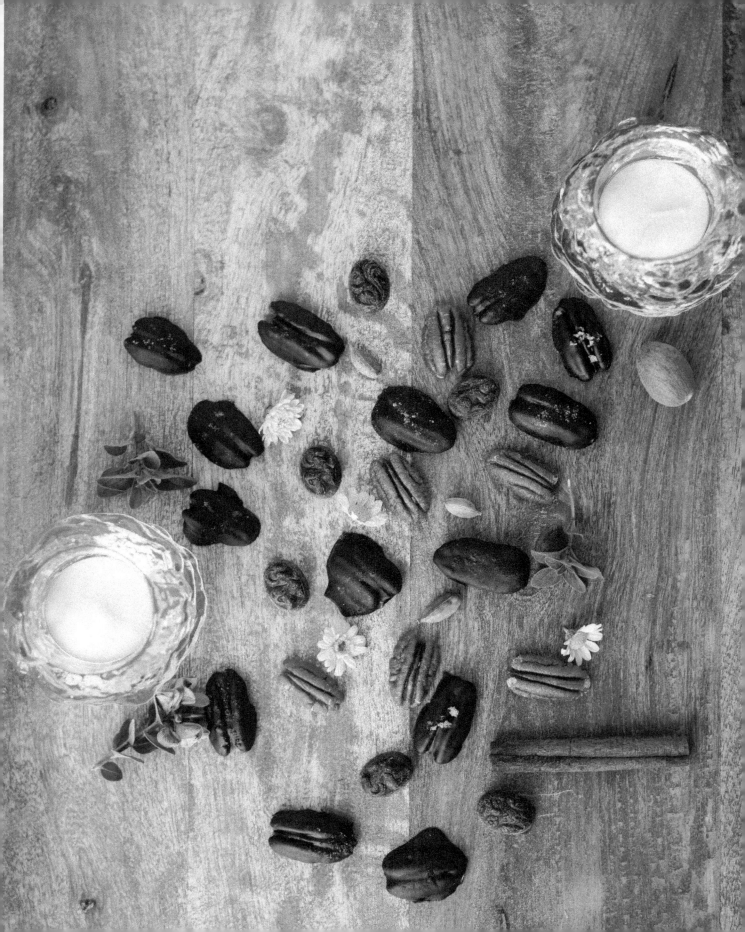

SPICED CHOCOLATE COVERED PECANS

Prep Time: 5 minutes
Cook Time: 25 minutes + 2 hours set time
Total Time: 30 minutes + 2 hours set time
Yield: 4 servings
Serving Size: approx. 10 pecans

INGREDIENTS

- 40-45 pecan halves (approx. 2.5 oz)
- 2 oz *(56 g)* 100% dark chocolate
- Spices of your choosing - my favorites were cinnamon, nutmeg, and salt

INSTRUCTIONS

1. Preheat oven to 350 F *(175 C)*.
2. Place the pecan halves in a single layer on some parchment paper and bake in oven for 7 minutes.
3. Let the pecan halves cool for 10-20 minutes.
4. Melt the dark chocolate (microwave on high for 2 minutes).
5. Dip each pecan half in the melted dark chocolate with a fork and place back on the parchment paper.
6. Sprinkle a small amount of the spice/salt of your choosing on top of the chocolate covered pecans.
7. Place in refrigerator for 1-2 hours to set.

Nutritional Data (estimates) - per serving:
Calories: 160   Fat: 15 g   Net Carbohydrates: 5 g   Protein: 3 g

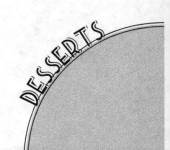

DESSERTS

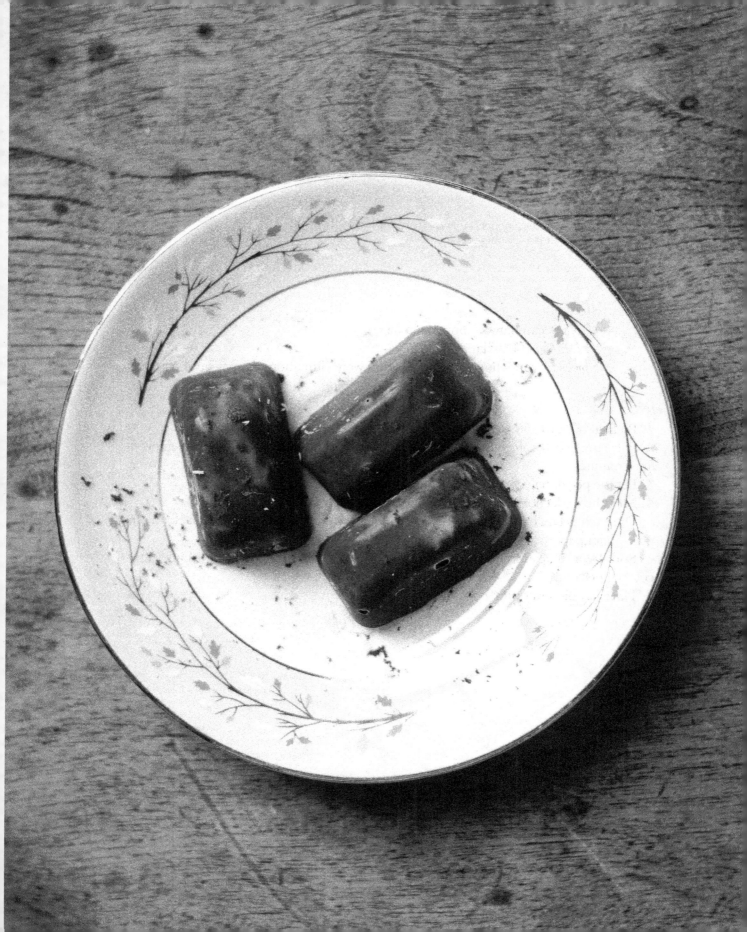

CHOCOLATE COFFEE COCONUT TRUFFLES

Prep Time: 10 minutes
Cook Time: 5 hours set time
Total Time: 10 minutes + 5 hours set time
Yield: 6 servings
Serving Size: 1 truffle

INGREDIENTS

- 1/2 cup *(120 g)* coconut butter (see page 183 for recipe)
- 3 Tablespoons *(15 g)* 100% cacao powder
- 1 Tablespoon *(5 g)* ground coffee beans
- 1 Tablespoon *(5 g)* unsweetened coconut flakes
- Dash of stevia (optional)
- 1 Tablespoon *(15 ml)* coconut oil

INSTRUCTIONS

1. Melt the coconut butter (in a microwave) so that it can be mixed with a fork.
2. Mix in all the ingredients (except the coconut oil) and mix well with a fork.
3. Take an ice-cube tray and pour approximately 1/4 teaspoon of coconut oil into 6 of the cups.
4. Spoon the mixture into each cup of the ice-cube tray and gently pat them flat with a fork.
5. Freeze for 4-5 hours.
6. Defrost at room temperature for 15-20 minutes before serving.

Nutritional Data (estimates) - per serving:
Calories: 160   Fat: 15 g   Net Carbohydrates: 3 g   Protein: 2 g

the Essential
KETO

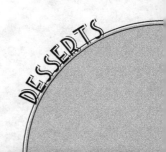

DESSERTS

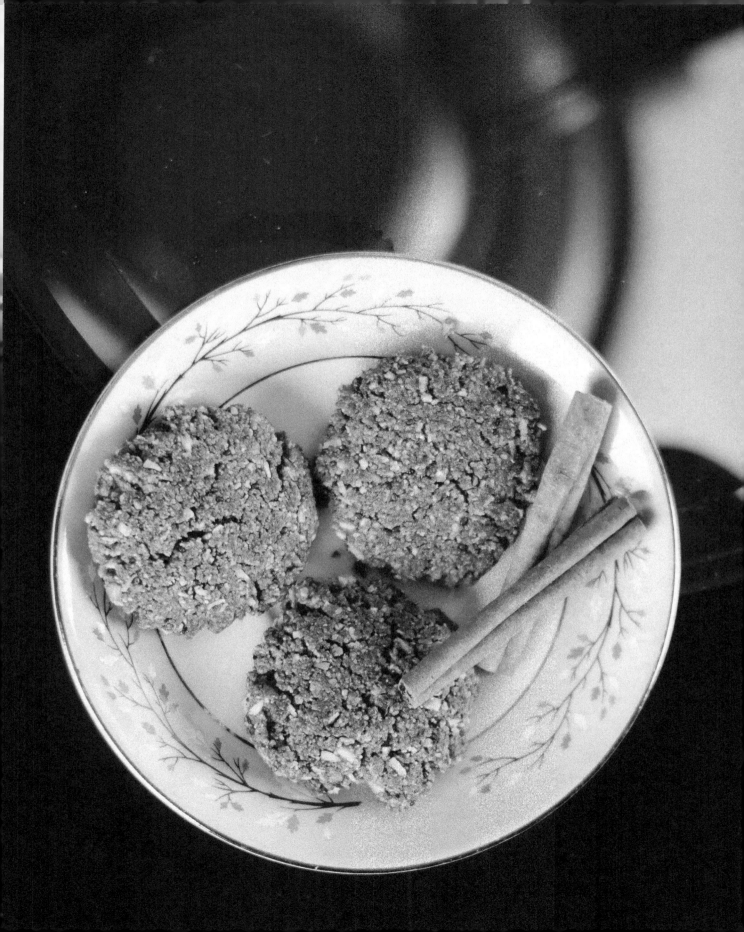

GINGER SPICE COOKIES

Prep Time: 10 minutes
Cook Time: 15 minutes
Total Time: 25 minutes
Yield: 12 servings
Serving Size: 1 cookie

INGREDIENTS

- 2 cups *(280 g)* whole almonds
- 2 Tablespoons *(80 g)* chia seeds
- 1/4 cup *(60 ml)* coconut oil
- 1 egg
- 3 Tablespoons *(15 g)* fresh ginger, grated
- 2 Tablespoons *(14 g)* cinnamon powder
- 1/2 teaspoon *(1 g)* nutmeg
- Stevia equivalent to 6 Tablespoons *(72 g)* of sugar
- Dash of salt

INSTRUCTIONS

1. Preheat oven to 350 F *(175 C)*.
2. Food process or blend the whole almonds with the chia seeds.
3. Mix all the ingredients together in a large bowl.
4. Form 12 small cookies with your hands and place on a baking tray lined with parchment paper.
5. Bake at 350 F for 15 minutes.

If you're looking to make desserts, then stevia is a good option for sweeteners, but try not to eat too much desserts as it can make it harder for you to give up sweets.

Nutritional Data (estimates) - per serving:
Calories: 200   Fat: 18 g   Net Carbohydrates: 3 g   Protein: 6 g

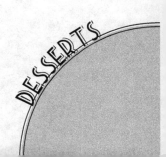

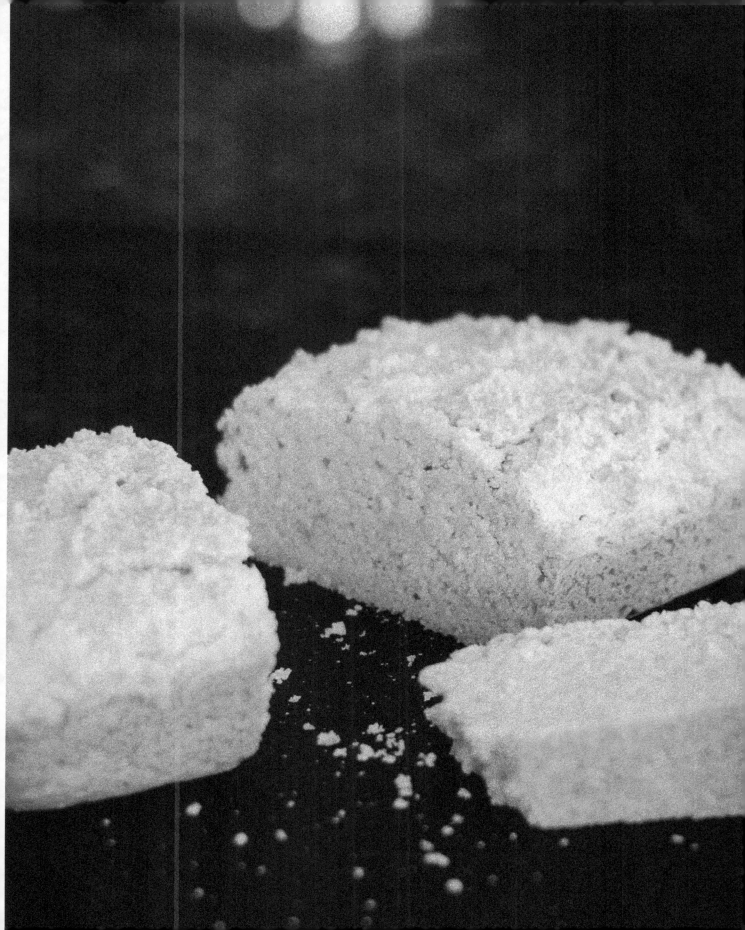

FRESHLY BAKED LOAF OF BREAD

Prep Time: 10 minutes
Cook Time: 1 hour
Total Time: 1 hour 10 minutes
Yield: 8 servings
Serving Size: 1 slice

INGREDIENTS

- 3 cups *(330g)* almond flour
- 1/2 cup + 2 Tablespoons *(150 ml)* coconut oil
- 1/4 cup *(60 ml)* coconut milk
- 3 eggs
- 2 teaspoons *(9 g)* baking powder
- 1 teaspoon *(5 g)* baking soda
- 1 Tablespoon *(3 g)* Italian seasoning
- 1/4 teaspoon *(1 g)* salt

INSTRUCTIONS

1. Preheat oven to 300 F *(150 C)*.
2. Grease a loaf pan *(9 in by 5 in (22.5 cm by 12.5 cm))* with olive oil or coconut oil.
3. Mix together all ingredients in a large bowl.
4. Pour the batter into the pan and spread it out so that it fills the pan evenly.
5. Bake for 60 minutes.
6. Let cool, flip pan, and cut into slices with a bread knife.

Nutritional Data (estimates) - per serving:
Calories: 400   Fat: 41 g   Net Carbohydrates: 5 g   Protein: 11 g

the Essential
KETO
COOKBOOK

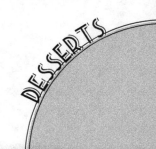

DESSERTS

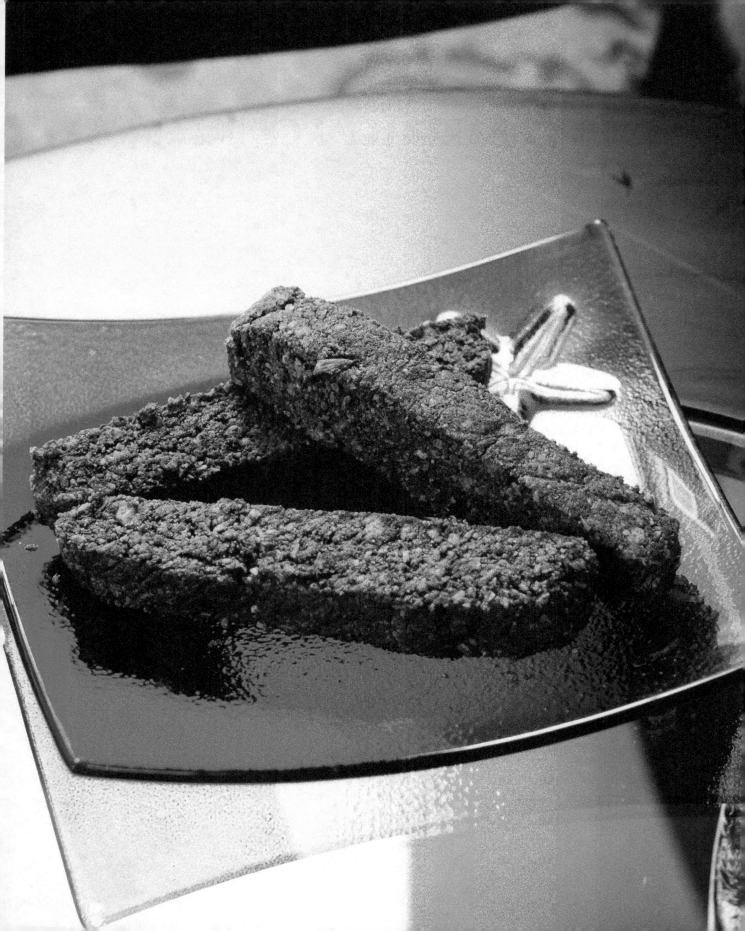

CHOCOLATE BISCOTTI

Prep Time: 10 minutes
Cook Time: 12 minutes
Total Time: 22 minutes
Yield: 8 servings
Serving Size: 1 slice

INGREDIENTS

- 2 cups *(280 g)* whole almonds
- 2 Tablespoons *(80 g)* chia seeds
- 1/4 cup *(20 g)* unsweetened shredded coconut
- 1 egg
- 1/4 cup *(60 ml)* coconut oil
- 1/4 cup *(20 g)* cacao powder
- Pinch of stevia
- 1/4 teaspoon *(1 g)* salt
- 1 teaspoon *(4 g)* baking soda

INSTRUCTIONS

1. Preheat oven to 350 F *(175 C)*.
2. Food process or blend the whole almonds with the chia seeds (the mixture should be fairly fine).
3. Mix all the ingredients together well.
4. Place the dough on a piece of aluminum foil to shape into 8 biscotti-shaped slices (long thin fingers). (Or you could refrigerate the dough for 30 minutes in a loaf shape and then carefully slice it.)
5. Bake at 350 F for 12 minutes.
6. Turn the oven temperature down to 300 F *(150 C)* and bake for another 15 minutes. Let cool to harden.

Nutritional Data (estimates) - per serving:
Calories: 350   Fat: 30 g   Net Carbohydrates: 5 g   Protein: 10 g

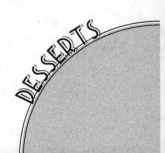

CUCUMBER LIME GUMMIES

Prep Time: 10 minutes
Cook Time: 5 minutes + 2 hours set time
Total Time: 15 minutes + 2 hours set time
Yield: 3-4 servings
Serving Size: 4 small gummies

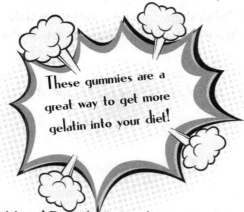

INGREDIENTS

- 1 cucumber, peeled (*approx 1/2 lb or 225 g*)
- 15-20 fresh mint leaves
  (or 1 Tablespoon *(3 g)* mint tea leaves)
- Juice from 1/2 lime
- 1.5 Tablespoons *(10 g)* gelatin powder
- Dash of stevia (optional)

INSTRUCTIONS

1. In a blender, blend the cucumber, mint leaves, lime juice, and stevia.
2. Strain the mixture and place the liquid (approx. 1/2 cup or 120 ml liquid) into a small pot on the stove.
3. Heat on medium heat until the liquid starts to simmer.
4. Stir in the gelatin powder (adding a small amount at a time) until it's all dissolved. Strain again to remove any lumps that might have formed.
5. Pour into silicone molds (ice cube trays work well) and refrigerate for 2 hours.

These gummies are a great way to get more gelatin into your diet!

Nutritional Data (estimates) - per serving:
Calories: 10   Fat: 0 g   Net Carbohydrates: 0 g   Protein: 2 g

the Essential
KETO

CHOCOLATE CHIA PUDDING

Prep Time: 5 minutes
Cook Time: 8 hours set time
Total Time: 5 minutes + 8 hours set time
Yield: 2 servings
Serving Size: 1 cup

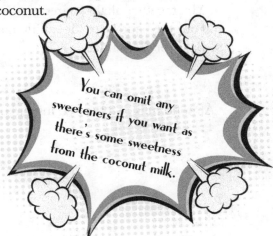

INGREDIENTS

- 2 Tablespoons *(10 g)* unsweetened cacao powder
- 1 cup *(240 ml)* unsweetened coconut milk
- 1/3 cup *(215 g)* chia seeds
- 1 Tablespoon *(5 g)* unsweetened shredded coconut (for topping)
- Spices and/or sweetener of choice

INSTRUCTIONS

1. Mix together all the ingredients (cacao powder, coconut milk, chia seeds, spices, and sweetener) in a bowl.
2. Cover the bowl and refrigerate overnight (approx. 8 hours).
3. Blend the mixture until smooth (this helped to get all the cacao powder nicely mixed in). Pour into cups and top with shredded coconut.

You can omit any sweeteners if you want as there's some sweetness from the coconut milk.

Nutritional Data (estimates) - per serving:
Calories: 300   Fat: 24 g   Net Carbohydrates: 3 g   Protein: 8 g

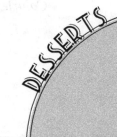

DESSERTS

JALAPEÑO "CORN" BREAD

Prep Time: 10 minutes
Cook Time: 20 minutes
Total Time: 30 minutes
Yield: 6 servings
Serving Size: 2 muffins

INGREDIENTS

- 3/4 cup *(83 g)* almond flour
- 1/4 cup *(28 g)* coconut flour
- 2 teaspoons *(9 g)* baking powder
- 1 teaspoon *(5 g)* salt
- Very small dash of stevia
- 3 eggs
- 1/2 cup *(120 ml)* coconut milk
- 3 jalapeño peppers, diced
- Coconut oil for greasing muffin pan or use muffin liners

INSTRUCTIONS

1. Preheat oven to 350 F *(175 C)*.
2. Grease muffin pan with coconut oil or use muffin liners.
3. Mix together all the ingredients well in a large bowl.
4. Pour the batter into the muffin pan.
5. Bake for 20 minutes.

SUBSTITUTIONS

- Almond milk can be used instead of coconut milk.

Nutritional Data (estimates) - per serving:
Calories: 150   Fat: 15 g   Net Carbohydrates: 2 g   Protein: 5 g

the Essential
KETO

BLACK & WHITE LAYERED PEPPERMINT PATTIES

Prep Time: 15 minutes
Cook Time: 3 hours set time
Total Time: 15 minutes + 3 hours set time
Yield: 24 patties
Serving Size: 1 patty

INGREDIENTS

For the white layers:
- ½ cup *(120 g)* coconut butter
- ¼ cup *(20 g)* unsweetened shredded coconut
- 2 Tablespoons *(30 ml)* coconut oil
- 1 teaspoon *(5 ml)* peppermint extract (add more to taste)
- Stevia to taste (optional)

For the black layers:
- 4 oz *(115 g)* 100% dark chocolate
- 4 Tablespoons *(60 ml)* coconut oil

INSTRUCTIONS

1. To make the white layers, soften the coconut butter and the 2 tablespoons of coconut oil and mix them together with the unsweetened shredded coconut, stevia, and peppermint extract.
2. Spoon 2 teaspoons of the white mixture into each mini muffin cup and refrigerate for 1 hour to set. Check this layer is solid before proceeding to the next step. If you don't have a mini muffin tray, then use a regular muffin tray - serving size will be half of a patty.
3. To make the black layers, melt the 4 tablespoons of coconut oil and the 4 oz dark chocolate and combine together well. Spoon 1 teaspoon of the black mixture into each mini muffin cup so that it forms a thin layer above the already solid white layer. Set in fridge for 1 hour. Check this layer is solid before going to the next step.
4. Repeat steps 2 and 3 for as many layers as you want.

Nutritional Data (estimates) - per serving:
Calories: 100   Fat: 10 g   Net Carbohydrates: 2 g   Protein: 1 g

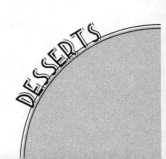

SALTED PRETZEL BITES

Prep Time: 15 minutes
Cook Time: 15 minutes
Total Time: 30 minutes
Yield: 4 servings
Serving Size: 7 pretzel bites *(approx.)*

INGREDIENTS

- 3 eggs
- 1.5 cups *(165 g)* almond flour
- 2 Tablespoons *(30 ml)* ghee, melted
- 3 Tablespoons *(21 g)* coconut flour
- 1/2 teaspoon *(3 g)* salt
- 1 egg, whisked *(as egg wash)*
- Coarse sea salt for sprinkling *(optional)*

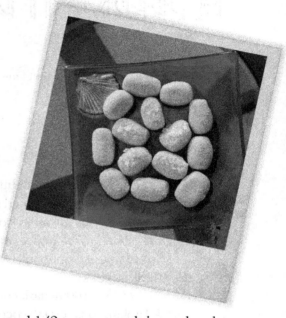

INSTRUCTIONS

1. Preheat oven to 350 F *(175 C)*.
2. Place 3 eggs, almond flour, ghee, coconut flour, and 1/2 teaspoon salt into a bowl and mix well until it forms a dough.
3. Let the dough sit for 5 minutes.
4. Roll into pretzel bites *(small balls)* and place on a parchment paper lined baking tray.
5. Bake in oven for 6-7 minutes.
6. Take the pretzels out and heat oven to 400 F *(200 C)*.
7. Turn each pretzel bite over, brush some of the whisked egg onto the top, and sprinkle some of the coarse sea salt on them.
8. Bake for 5 more minutes.

Nutritional Data (estimates) - per serving:
Calories: 320   Fat: 28 g   Net Carbohydrates: 4 g   Protein: 13 g

SAVORY ITALIAN CRACKERS

Prep Time: 15 minutes
Cook Time: 10 minutes
Total Time: 25 minutes
Yield: 4 servings
Serving Size: 5 crackers *(approx.)*

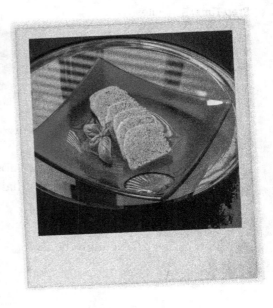

INGREDIENTS

- 1.5 cups *(165 g)* almond flour
- 1 egg
- 2 Tablespoons *(30 ml)* olive oil
- 3/4 teaspoon *(4 g)* salt
- 1/4 teaspoon *(0.5 g)* basil
- 1/2 teaspoon *(1 g)* thyme
- 1/4 teaspoon *(0.5 g)* oregano
- 1/2 teaspoon *(1 g)* onion powder
- 1/4 teaspoon *(0.5 g)* garlic powder

INSTRUCTIONS

1. Preheat oven to 350 F *(175 C)*.
2. Mix all the ingredients well to form a dough.
3. Shape dough into a long rectangular log (use some foil or cling film to pack the dough tight) and then cut into thin slices *(approximately 0.2 inches (0.5 cm) thick)*. Gently place each slice onto a parchment paper lined baking tray. It makes approx. 20-30 crackers, depending on size.
4. Bake for 10-12 minutes.

SUBSTITUTIONS

• Italian seasoning (see page 177 for recipe) can be used instead of basil, thyme, oregano, onion powder, and garlic powder if you don't have those available.
• Other nut flours can be used instead of almond flour (just food process the nuts using a food processor or blender into a fine meal).

Nutritional Data (estimates) - per serving:
Calories: 280   Fat: 25 g   Net Carbohydrates: 3 g   Protein: 9 g

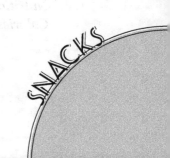

SNACKS

KETO SUPERFOODS TRAIL MIX

Prep Time: 5 minutes
Cook Time: 0 minutes
Total Time: 5 minutes
Yield: 1 serving
Serving Size: 1 small bowl

Make a large batch and keep in airtight container to enjoy as a quick snack!

INGREDIENTS

- 5 freeze-dried berries (I used raspberries)
- 2 Brazil nuts
- 2 Tablespoons *(28 g)* cacao nibs
- 1 Tablespoon *(3 g)* coconut flakes

INSTRUCTIONS

1. Mix together all the ingredients.

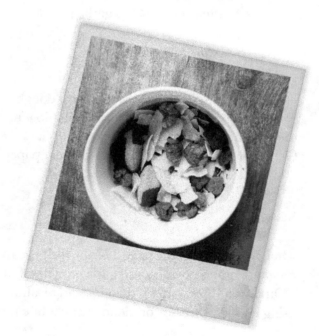

Nutritional Data (estimates) - per serving:
Calories: 280   Fat: 25 g   Net Carbohydrates: 1 g   Protein: 2 g

CRUNCHY KALE CHIPS

Prep Time: 5 minutes
Cooking Time: varies *(depending on cooking method)*
Total Time: varies *(depending on cooking method)*
Yield: 2 servings
Serving Size: 1 bowl

INGREDIENTS

- 4 large kale leaves
- 1/2 Tablespoon *(7 g)* salt
- 2 Tablespoons *(30 ml)* olive oil
- 1/4 Tablespoon *(1 g)* crushed
  red pepper *(optional)*
- 1/2 Tablespoon *(3 g)* paprika *(optional)*

Kale chips are a great crunchy snack, and there are lots of different ways to make them. The dehydrator method is the best, but the oven and microwave also work.

INSTRUCTIONS

1. Wash the kale leaves and remove the stems so you're just left with the leaves. Dry the leaves well.
2. In a bowl, add the leaves and the salt, olive oil, and spices. Mix well.
3. If using the oven, preheat oven to 300 F *(150 C)* and place the leaves flat on a baking tray *(with no overlapping)*. Bake for 5-10 minutes - make sure the leaves get crispy but are not burnt.
4. If using a dehydrator, place the leaves flat on the dehydrator trays *(with no overlapping)* and dehydrate until crispy on 135 F *(57 C)* *(for 3-5 hours)*.
5. If using a microwave, place the leaves on a microwavable plate and place in microwave on full power for 2-3 minutes *(check after 2 minutes to make sure they aren't burning - you may need to test the time and power for your microwave settings)*.

Nutritional Data (estimates) - per serving:
Calories: 170   Fat: 14 g   Net Carbohydrates: 6 g   Protein: 4 g

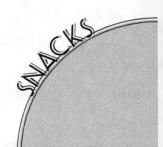

CONDIMENTS, SEASONING & SAUCES

CHAPTER 6

HOMEMADE ITALIAN SEASONING

Prep Time: 5 minutes
Cook Time: 0 minutes
Total Time: 5 minutes
Yield: 1 cup
Serving Size: N/A

INGREDIENTS

- 1/4 cup *(12 g)* dried basil
- 1/4 cup *(12 g)* dried rosemary
- 1/4 cup *(12 g)* dried thyme
- 1/4 cup *(12 g)* dried oregano
- 1 Tablespoon *(10 g)* garlic powder
- 1 Tablespoon *(7 g)* onion powder

INSTRUCTIONS

1. Mix all the ingredients together well and store in an airtight container.

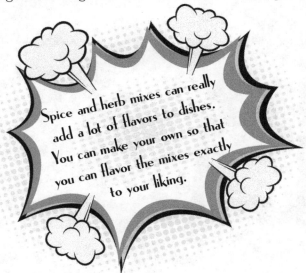

Spice and herb mixes can really add a lot of flavors to dishes. You can make your own so that you can flavor the mixes exactly to your liking.

Nutritional Data (estimates) - per tablespoon:
Calories: 10   Fat: 0 g   Net Carbohydrates: 1 g   Protein: 0 g

the Essential
KETO
COOKBOOK

CONDIMENTS

GARLIC SAUCE

Prep Time: 5 minutes
Cook Time: 0 minutes
Total Time: 5 minutes
Yield: approx. 1.5 cups
Serving Size: N/A

Pair this sauce with any meal to instantly make your meal more tasty.

INGREDIENTS

- 1 head garlic, peeled
- 1 teaspoon *(5 g)* salt
- Approx. 1/4 cup *(60 ml)* lemon juice
- Approx. 1 cup *(240 ml)* olive oil

INSTRUCTIONS

1. Place the garlic cloves and salt into the blender. Then add in around 1/8 cup of the lemon juice and 1/2 cup of olive oil.
2. Blend well for 5-10 seconds, then slow your blender down and drizzle in more lemon juice and olive oil alternatively until a creamy consistency forms.

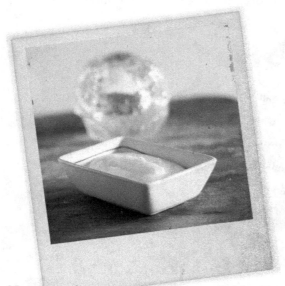

Nutritional Data (estimates) - per tablespoon:
Calories: 80   Fat: 9 g   Net Carbohydrates: 0 g   Protein: 0 g

CAESAR DRESSING

Prep Time: 15 minutes
Cook Time: 0 minutes
Total Time: 15 minutes
Yield: approx. 1.5 cups
Serving Size: N/A

INGREDIENTS

- 2 egg yolks
- 1/4 cup *(60 ml)* apple cider vinegar
- 1 cup *(240 ml)* coconut oil, melted
- 6 anchovies
- 2 teaspoons *(9 g)* Dijon mustard
- 2 large cloves of garlic, minced
- 1/4 teaspoon *(1 g)* salt
- 1/4 teaspoon *(1 g)* freshly ground black pepper

INSTRUCTIONS

1. Blend or whisk the 2 egg yolks with the apple cider vinegar.
2. Slowly add in the coconut oil while blending until it forms a mayo texture.
3. Add in rest of the oil, the anchovies, mustard, garlic, salt, and pepper and blend well.

Most store-bought salad dressings use unhealthy oils like canola and sunflower oil - they can be inflammatory due to the way they're processed. So, best to make your own so you can make sure they're tasty and healthy.

Nutritional Data (estimates) - per tablespoon:
Calories: 80   Fat: 9 g   Net Carbohydrates: 0 g   Protein: 0 g

CONDIMENTS

CAJUN SEASONING

Prep Time: 5 minutes
Cook Time: 0 minutes
Total Time: 5 minutes
Yield: 6 Tablespoons
Serving Size: N/A

INGREDIENTS

- 1.5 Tablespoons *(10 g)* paprika
- 1.5 Tablespoons *(15 g)* garlic powder
- 1/2 Tablespoons *(3 g)* onion powder
- 1/2 Tablespoons *(2 g)* black pepper
- 1 teaspoon *(2 g)* cayenne pepper
- 1 teaspoon *(2 g)* dried oregano
- 1 teaspoon *(1 g)* dried thyme
- 1 teaspoon *(1 g)* dried basil
- 1-2 teaspoons *(5-10 g)* of salt *(to taste)*

INSTRUCTIONS

1. Mix all the dried spices and herbs together and store in an airtight jar.

You can use this as a rub on your meats before adding them to your slow cooker or before grilling them. Just make sure to add less cayenne pepper if you don't like spicy food.

Nutritional Data (estimates) - per tablespoon:
Calories: 15   Fat: 0 g   Net Carbohydrates: 2 g   Protein: 0 g

COCONUT MAYONNAISE

Prep Time: 15 minutes
Cook Time: 0 minutes
Total Time: 15 minutes
Yield: approx. 1.5 cups
Serving Size: N/A

INGREDIENTS

- 2 egg yolks
- 2 Tablespoons *(30 ml)* of apple cider vinegar
- 1 cup *(240 ml)* coconut oil, melted *(but not too hot)*

INSTRUCTIONS

1. Blend or whisk the 2 egg yolks with the 2 Tablespoons *(30 ml)* of apple cider vinegar.
2. Slowly add in the coconut oil while blending *(I used a blender and added in the coconut oil from the hole at top of the blender approximately 1/2 tablespoon at a time until it forms a mayo texture).*
3. Add in rest of the oil (and a bit more if you want a less thick texture) and blend well.
4. Use immediately *(if you want to store it in the fridge, then use 1/2 cup olive oil or avocado oil and 1/2 cup coconut oil instead of only coconut oil, as the coconut oil will make the mayo solidify in the fridge).*
We try to use it within a week.

SUBSTITUTIONS

- Olive oil or avocado oil can be used instead of coconut oil.
- Spices and herbs can be added for different types of mayo.
- Lemon juice can be used instead of apple cider vinegar (but it gives a different taste to the mayo).

Nutritional Data (estimates) - per tablespoon:
Calories: 80   Fat: 9 g   Net Carbohydrates: 0 g   Protein: 0 g

the Essential
KETO
cookbook

CONDIMENTS

COCONUT RANCH DRESSING

Prep Time: 10 minutes
Cook Time: 0 minutes
Total Time: 10 minutes
Yield: approx. 1/2 cup
Serving Size: N/A

INGREDIENTS

- 1/4 cup *(60 ml)* of mayo (see page 181 for recipe)
- 1/4 cup *(60 ml)* coconut milk
- 1 clove of garlic, minced
- 1/2 teaspoon *(1 g)* onion powder
- 1 Tablespoon *(4 g)* fresh parsley, finely chopped *(or 1 tsp (0.5 g) dried parsley)*
- 1 Tablespoon *(3 g)* fresh chives, finely chopped *(or omit)*
- 1 teaspoon *(1 g)* fresh dill, finely chopped *(or 1/2 tsp (0.5 g) dried dill)*
- Dash of salt
- Dash of pepper

INSTRUCTIONS

1. Mix together the mayo, coconut milk, onion powder, salt, and pepper with a fork.
2. Gently mix in the garlic and fresh herbs.

This ranch dressing goes great with the fiery buffalo wings (see page 50 for recipe).

Nutritional Data (estimates) - per tablespoon:
Calories: 50   Fat: 6 g   Net Carbohydrates: 0 g   Protein: 0 g

HOMEMADE COCONUT BUTTER

Prep Time: 10 minutes
Cook Time: 0 minutes
Total Time: 10 minutes
Yield: approx. 3 cups
Serving Size: N/A

If you can't buy coconut butter, then use this recipe to make it yourself. It tastes great spread on some 100% dark chocolate for a quick snack.

INGREDIENTS

- 6 cups *(480 g)* of unsweetened shredded coconut (or coconut flakes or coconut powder)
- 2 Tablespoons *(15 ml)* coconut oil, melted (if not using the VitaMix with a tamper or a Blendtec with the twister jar)

INSTRUCTIONS

1. Add the shredded coconut to the blender or food processor and blend on high.
2. If using the VitaMix with a tamper or a Blendtec with the twister jar, push the coconut down while you blend. Otherwise, stop the blender and push the coconut down with a spoon, and repeat 3 times.
3. If not using a VitaMix or a Blendtec, add the melted coconut oil in and blend on high for 10 minutes.

Nutritional Data (estimates) - per tablespoon:
Calories: 60   Fat: 6 g   Net Carbohydrates: 1 g   Protein: 1 g

CONDIMENTS

SLOW COOKER GHEE

Prep Time: 0 minutes
Cook Time: 3 hours
Total Time: 3 hours
Yield: 2 cups
Serving Size: N/A

INGREDIENTS
- 16 oz *(454 g)* butter

INSTRUCTIONS
1. Place butter into slow cooker and place lid on (slightly ajar so that the steam escapes).
2. Turn slow cooker on low for 2-3 hours until milk solids brown and fall to the bottom and bubbles slow down.
3. Place the cheesecloth at the top of the funnel and the funnel end into the mason jar.
4. Pour ghee through the cheesecloth through the funnel into the mason jar.
5. Store in fridge.

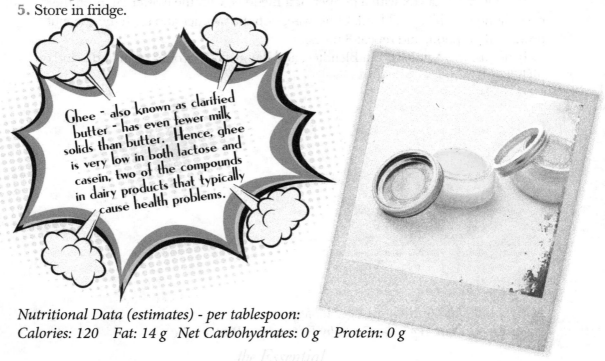

Ghee - also known as clarified butter - has even fewer milk solids than butter. Hence, ghee is very low in both lactose and casein, two of the compounds in dairy products that typically cause health problems.

Nutritional Data (estimates) - per tablespoon:
Calories: 120   Fat: 14 g   Net Carbohydrates: 0 g   Protein: 0 g

the Essential
KETO

CHINESE CHILI OIL

Prep Time: 5 minutes
Cook Time: 15 minutes
Total Time: 20 minutes
Yield: 1 cup of sauce
Serving Size: N/A

INGREDIENTS
- 3.5 oz *(100 g)* dried red Chinese or Thai chili peppers
- 2 Tablespoons *(15 g)* of Szechuan peppercorns
- 1 cup *(240 ml)* coconut oil

INSTRUCTIONS
1. Food process the dried red peppers and the Szechuan peppercorns together.
2. Heat the coconut oil in a pan on medium heat and put the food processed spices in.
3. Watch for the oil to start bubbling and then cook for an extra 3-5 minutes until the peppercorn pieces start to turn a bit darker (don't let them turn too dark or else they'll burn).
4. Place in a glass container and store.

Add this sauce into your sautes for an extra spicy kick to your dishes. Or it you steam vegetables, then just mix a small amount of this oil with some tamari sauce with the vegetables to take the blandness out of them.

Nutritional Data (estimates) - per tablespoon:
Calories: 80   Fat: 9 g   Net Carbohydrates: 0 g   Protein: 0 g

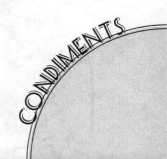

CASHEW CHEESE

Prep Time: 10 minutes
Cook Time: 0 minutes
Total Time: 10 minutes
Yield: 1 cup
Serving Size: N/A

INGREDIENTS

- 1/2 cup *(70 g)* raw cashews, soaked overnight
- 1 Tablespoon *(15 ml)* coconut oil
- 1/2 cup *(120 ml)* water

INSTRUCTIONS

1. Place the raw cashews into a bowl of room temperature water so that it covers the cashews, drape a paper towel or tea towel over the bowl to prevent dust settling, and soak overnight.
2. Place the soaked cashews, 1/2 cup fresh water, and coconut oil into a blender and blend until smooth.

Nutritional Data (estimates) - per tablespoon:
Calories: 25   Fat: 2 g   Net Carbohydrates: 1 g   Protein: 1 g

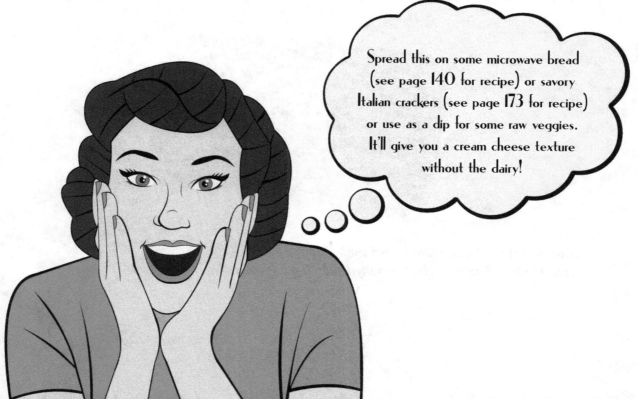

Spread this on some microwave bread (see page 140 for recipe) or savory Italian crackers (see page 173 for recipe) or use as a dip for some raw veggies. It'll give you a cream cheese texture without the dairy!

EASY GUACAMOLE

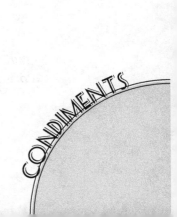

Prep Time: 10 minutes
Cooking Time: 0 minutes
Total Time: 10 minutes
Yield: 1 cup
Serving Size: N/A

INGREDIENTS

- 2 ripe avocados
- 1 small tomato, diced
- 1/4 cup *(8 g)* cilantro, finely chopped
- Juice from half a lime
- Salt to taste
- 1 jalapeño, finely chopped *(optional)*
- 1/2 teaspoon *(1 g)* chili powder *(optional)*
- 1 teaspoon *(3 g)* garlic powder *(optional)*
- 1 teaspoon *(2g)* onion powder *(optional)*

INSTRUCTIONS

1. Cut the avocados in half, remove the stone in the middle, and scoop out the flesh into a bowl.
2. Mash up the avocado flesh using a spoon or fork.
3. Add in the tomatoes, cilantro, lime juice, salt to taste, jalapeño, chili powder, garlic powder, and onion powder.
4. Mix well.

> Guacamole is a quick and easy condiment to make and goes great with meats, eggs, and vegetables.

Nutritional Data (estimates) - per tablespoon:
Calories: 40   Fat: 4 g   Net Carbohydrates: 1 g   Protein: 1 g

CONDIMENTS

OREGANO RASPBERRY LIVER PATE

Prep Time: 10 minutes
Cooking Time: 20 minutes
Total Time: 30 minutes
Yield: 4 servings
Serving Size: 2-3 Tablespoons *(approx.)*

INGREDIENTS

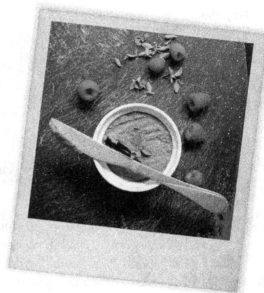

- 0.7 lb *(317 g)* chicken liver
- 2 Tablespoons *(30 ml)* ghee
  (may need extra)
- 1/2 onion, chopped
- Approx. 50 oregano leaves
- 10 raspberries (optional)
  - makes the pate less smooth
- Salt to taste

INSTRUCTIONS

1. Melt 2 Tablespoons of ghee in a pan and saute the chopped onions and chicken liver until the liver is cooked (just pink inside). This takes 10-15 minutes on medium heat, and you may find putting a lid onto the pan for 5 minutes at the end helps.
2. Add in the oregano leaves a few minutes before the liver is done.
3. Blend the liver, onions, oregano, raspberries, and salt until smooth (add in an extra tablespoon of ghee if needed to make the pate smoother).

SUBSTITUTIONS

- Other herbs and spices can be used instead of the oregano and raspberries.

This goes really well with the savory Italian crackers (see page 173 for recipe).

Nutritional Data (estimates) - per serving:
Calories: 180   Fat: 11 g   Net Carbohydrates: 3 g   Protein: 15 g

the Essential
KETO

DRINKS AND BROTHS

CHAPTER 7

EASY BONE BROTH

Prep Time: 5 minutes
Cook Time: 10 hours
Total Time: 10 hours 5 minutes
Yield: 8-16 servings *(depends on size of crockpot)*
Serving Size: 1 cup *(approx.)*

> After you've made the first batch of broth, you can make additional batches with the same bones. Typically, bones will last for at least 4-5 batches of broth.

INGREDIENTS

- 3-4 lbs *(1.5-2 kg)* of bones *(I typically use beef bones)*
- 1 gallon *(4 l)* water *(adjust for your slow cooker size)*
- 2 Tablespoons *(30 ml)* apple cider vinegar or lemon juice

INSTRUCTIONS

1. Add everything to the slow cooker and cook on the low setting for 10 hours.
2. Cool the broth, then strain and pour broth into a container.
3. Store the broth in the refrigerator or freezer until you're ready to use it.
4. Scoop out the congealed fat on top of the broth *(optional, but the broth is otherwise very fatty)*.
5. Heat broth when needed *(with spices, vegetables, etc.)*.

Nutritional Data (estimates) - per serving:
Calories: 80   Fat: 2 g   Net Carbohydrates: 0 g   Protein: 12 g

> There are tons of variations you can make - try adding in onions, ginger, and carrots into the slow cooker as well.

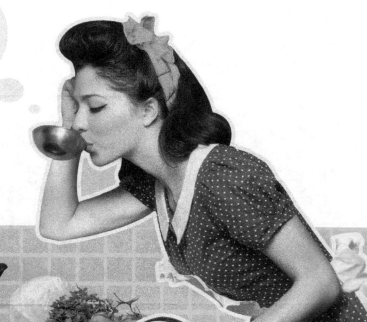

SINH TO BO (VIETNAMESE SMOOTHIE)

Prep Time: 5 minutes
Cook Time: 0 minutes
Total Time: 5 minutes
Yield: 2 servings
Serving Size: 1 glass

INGREDIENTS

- 1 avocado
- 1 cup *(500 g)* ice
- 1/2 cup *(120 ml)* coconut milk - add a little bit more if you have trouble getting the mixture to blend
- Stevia to taste (optional)

Traditionally, this is made using condensed milk, but I've used coconut milk instead to make this dairy-free and sugar-free.

INSTRUCTIONS

1. Cut a ripe avocado in half.
2. Use a spoon to scoop out the avocado flesh.
3. Place the avocado flesh into the blender with the ice and coconut milk (and stevia), and blend well (start slow and increase the speed slowly).
4. Add more coconut milk if necessary to blend until smooth.

SUBSTITUTIONS

- Almond milk can be used instead of coconut milk.

Nutritional Data (estimates) - per serving:
Calories: 300   Fat: 30 g   Net Carbohydrates: 2 g   Protein: 3 g

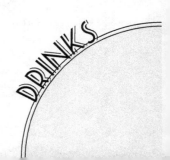
DRINKS

COCONUT MASALA CHAI

Prep Time: 5 minutes
Cook Time: 5 minutes
Total Time: 10 minutes
Yield: 2 servings
Serving Size: 1 cup

INGREDIENTS

- 1 cup *(240 ml)* coconut milk
- 1 cup *(240 ml)* water
- Stevia to taste (optional)
- 1 Tablespoon *(2 g)* loose black tea leaves
- Pinch of masala tea spice blend *(recipe below)*

Masala tea spice blend:
- 1 Tablespoon *(7 g)* nutmeg
- 1 Tablespoon *(5 g)* ginger powder
- 1 Tablespoon *(6 g)* cardamom
- 1 Tablespoon *(5 g)* black pepper
- 1 Tablespoon *(8 g)* cinnamon
- 1 teaspoon *(2 g)* cloves
- 1 Tablespoon *(5 g)* dried basil *(optional)*, ground into a powder

INSTRUCTIONS

1. Heat the coconut milk and water in a saucepan.
2. Add in the stevia, the tea, and the spice blend. Mix well.
3. Heat at a low simmer for approx. 4-5 minutes.
4. Taste the tea and add more sweetener or spices to taste.
5. Pour through a strainer *(to remove the tea leaves)* and serve immediately.

Nutritional Data (estimates) - per serving:
Calories: 300   Fat: 30 g   Net Carbohydrates: 2 g   Protein: 3 g

the Essential
KETO
COOKBOOK

GINGER BASIL TEA

Prep Time: 5 minutes
Cook Time: 0 minutes
Total Time: 5 minutes
Yield: 2 servings
Serving Size: 1 cup of tea

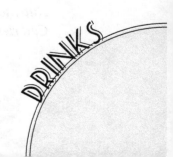

You can make a variety of herbal teas yourself - just pick your favorite herbs or berries and infuse them in hot water.

INGREDIENTS

- 2 cups *(480 ml)* boiling water
- 1/2 teaspoon *(1 g)* fresh ginger, grated *(or 10 very thin slices of ginger)*
- 4 fresh basil leaves

INSTRUCTIONS

1. Add the ginger and basil to a cup or teapot and pour boiling water into the cup/teapot.
2. Brew for 5 minutes.
3. Press the basil leaves gently with a spoon to get more flavor out of them, if desired.
4. Sieve out *(using a special teapot or a strainer)* the ginger and basil.
5. Enjoy hot or cold.

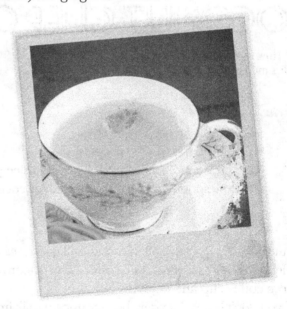

Nutritional Data (estimates) - per serving:
Calories: 0   Fat: 0 g   Net Carbohydrates: 0 g   Protein: 0 g

DRINKS

PUMPKIN SPICE LATTE

Total Time: 5 minutes
Yield: 1 cup of coffee

INGREDIENTS

- 1 cup *(240 ml)* black coffee
- 1 Tablespoon *(15 g)* pumpkin puree
- 1/4 teaspoon *(1 g)* cinnamon
- 1/4 teaspoon *(1 g)* nutmeg
- Dash of cloves
- 1 Tablespoon *(15 ml)* ghee

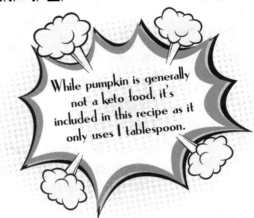

While pumpkin is generally not a keto food, it's included in this recipe as it only uses 1 tablespoon.

INSTRUCTIONS

1. Place all the ingredients into a blender and blend well for 15 seconds.

Nutritional Data (estimates) - per serving:
Calories: 120   Fat: 13 g   Net Carbohydrates: 1 g   Protein: 1 g

COCONUT GHEE COFFEE

Total Time: 5 minutes
Yield: 1 mug of coffee

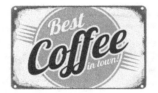

INGREDIENTS

- 1/2 Tablespoon *(7 g)* ghee
- 1/2 Tablespoon *(7 g)* coconut oil
- 1-2 cups *(240-480 ml)* of whatever coffee you like *(or black or rooibos tea)*
- 1 Tablespoon *(15 ml)* almond milk or coconut milk

INSTRUCTIONS

1. Put the ghee, coconut oil, almond milk *(or coconut milk)*, and the coffee into a blender.
2. Blend for 5-10 seconds. The coffee turns a foamy, creamy color. Pour it into your favorite coffee cup and enjoy!
3. If you don't have a blender, then try using a milk frother.

Nutritional Data (estimates) - per serving:
Calories: 150   Fat: 15 g   Net Carbohydrates: 0 g   Protein: 0 g

LEMON THYME INFUSED ICED TEA

Total Time: 10 minutes + overnight infusion
Yield: 6-8 cups of tea

Grow some herbs in your garden or on your kitchen windowsill. Fresh herbs are great for adding to dishes and are also perfect for making teas.

INGREDIENTS

- 4-6 cups *(1-1.5 l)* of black tea
- 6 sprigs of lemon thyme or other herb or spice

INSTRUCTIONS

1. Brew the black tea.
2. Remove the tea bag(s) and add 2 sprigs of lemon thyme into the hot tea.
3. Let cool and then refrigerate overnight.
4. Remove the lemon thyme and serve with ice and fresh sprigs of lemon thyme for decoration.

Nutritional Data (estimates) - per serving:
Calories: 0   Fat: 0 g   Net Carbohydrates: 0 g   Protein: 0 g

COCONUT ICED TEA LATTE

Total Time: 10 minutes
Yield: 2 cups of tea

INGREDIENTS

- 2 cups *(480 ml)* black tea
- 3 Tablespoons *(30 ml)* coconut milk (or to taste)
- Stevia to taste (optional)

Almond and coconut milk are great options for dairy-free milk. Just try to buy brands with as few added ingredients as possible. In particular, many brands of canned coconut milk don't have added ingredients.

INSTRUCTIONS

1. Brew the black tea.
2. Add in the coconut milk and stevia to taste.
3. Blend for a few seconds or use a milk frother.
4. Pour into a glass with ice.

Nutritional Data (estimates) - per cup:
Calories: 30   Fat: 3 g   Net Carbohydrates: 0 g   Protein: 0 g

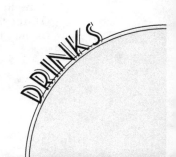
DRINKS

KETO MEAL PLAN

ABOUT THIS MEAL PLAN

This meal plan is designed for 2 people and covers breakfast, lunch, and dinner.

Important note: 1 batch means to make the recipe as stated, 2 batches means to make a double portion of the recipe.

WEEK 1

Day 1:
Breakfast: Make 1 batch of Kale and Chives Egg Muffins (page 27). Eat 2 muffins each and refrigerate the rest.
Lunch: Make 1 batch of Thai Chicken Pad See Ew (page 71).
Dinner: Make 1/2 batch of Spaghetti Squash Bolognese (page 92) with 1 batch of Creamy Cauliflower Mash (page 145). Use shredded zucchinis if you can't find spaghetti squash.

Day 2:
Breakfast: Reheat and eat rest of the premade Kale and Chives Egg Muffins.
Lunch: Make 1 batch of Turkey Arugula Salad (page 137).
Dinner: Make 1 batch of Beef Curry (page 100)) with 2 batches of Cauliflower White "Rice" (page 143). Eat 1/2 batch of beef curry with 1 batch of "rice" and refrigerate the rest.

Day 3:
Breakfast: Make 2 batches of Breakfast Turkey Wrap (page 29).
Lunch: Reheat and eat rest of the beef curry with "rice."
Dinner: Make 1 batch of Pan-Fried Pork Tenderloins (page 115) with 1/2 batch of Garlic Zucchini Saute (page 151).

Day 4:
Breakfast: Make 2 batches of Coconut Ghee Coffee (page 194).
Lunch: Make 1 batch of Basil Chicken Saute (page 78).
Dinner: Make 1/2 batch of Breaded Cod with Garlic Ghee Sauce (page 119) with 1 batch of Spinach Almond Saute (page 146).
Prep: Make 1 batch of Easy Bone Broth (page 190).

Day 5:
Breakfast: Make 4 batches of the Easy Seed & Nut Granola (page 35). Eat 1 serving each and save the rest in an airtight container.
Lunch: Make 1 batch of Italian Tuna Salad (page 47).
Dinner: Make 1 batch of Zucchini Beef Pho (page 87) using premade Easy Bone Broth.
Prep: Make 1 batch of Slow Cooker Oxtail Stew (page 133).

Day 6:
Breakfast: Make 2 batches of Almond Butter Chocolate Shake (page 32).
Lunch: Make 1 batch of Spinach Basil Chicken Meatballs (page 63).
Dinner: Premade Slow Cooker Oxtail Stew (2 servings) with 1/2 batch of Lemon Asparagus Saute with Bacon (page 147).

Day 7:
Breakfast: Make 1 batch of Spring Soup with Poached Egg (page 36) using premade Bone Broth.
Lunch: Make 1/2 batch of Guacamole Burger (page 95).
Dinner: Premade Slow Cooker Oxtail Stew (2 servings) with 1 batch of Cauliflower White "Rice" (page 143).

WEEK 2:

Day 1:
Breakfast: Eat the rest of the premade Easy Seed & Nut Granola.
Lunch: Make 1 batch of Easy Broccoli Beef Stir-Fry (page 102).
Dinner: Make 1 batch of Rosemary Baked Salmon (page 127) with 1/3 batch of Refreshing Cucumber Salad (page 150).
Prep: Make 1 batch of Tea Eggs (page 38).

Day 2:
Breakfast: Eat 2 premade Tea Eggs each.
Lunch: Make 1 batch of Liver and Onions (page 138).
Dinner: Make 1 batch of Mustard Ground Beef Saute (page 94).
Prep: Make 1 batch of Slow Cooker Bacon & Chicken (page 76).

Day 3:
Breakfast: Eat 2 premade Tea Eggs each.
Lunch: Make 1 batch of Big Easy Salad (page 57).
Dinner: Premade Slow Cooker Bacon & Chicken (2 servings) with 1/3 batch of Refreshing Cucumber Salad (page 150).

Day 4:
Breakfast: Eat 2 premade Tea Eggs each.
Lunch: Make 1 batch of Turkey Arugula Salad (page 137).
Dinner: Premade Slow Cooker Bacon & Chicken (2 servings) with 1 batch of Creamy Cauliflower Mash (page 145).

Day 5:
Breakfast: Make 2 batches of Coconut Ghee Coffee (page 194).
Lunch: Reheat and eat rest of the premade Slow Cooker Bacon & Chicken (2 servings).
Dinner: Make 1 batch of Cilantro Celery Salmon Stew (page 129) with 1 batch of Microwave Quick Bread (page 141).

Day 6:
Breakfast: Make 2 batches of Breakfast Green Smoothie (page 39).
Lunch: Make 2 batches of Easy Egg Drop Soup (page 52).
Dinner: Make 1/2 batch of Cumin Crusted Lamb Chops (page 134) with 1/2 batch of Lemon Asparagus Saute with Bacon (page 147).

Day 7:
Breakfast: Make 1 batch of Creamy Breakfast Porridge (page 25).
Lunch: Make 1 batch of Chicken Noodle Soup (page 43).
Dinner: Make 1 batch of Mu Shu Pork (page 113).

KETOGENIC DIET FOOD LIST

VEGETABLES

Try to stick to green leafy vegetables and avoid root vegetables to keep your daily carbohydrate intake low.

Arugula (Rocket)
Artichokes
Asparagus
Bell Peppers
Bok Choy
Broccoli
Brussels Sprouts
Butterhead Lettuce
Cabbage
Carrots (not too much)
Cauliflower
Celery
Chard
Chicory Greens
Chives
Cucumber
Dandelion Greens
Eggplant (Aubergine)
Endives

Fennel
Garlic
Jicama
Kale
Kohlrabi
Leeks
Leafy Greens (Various Kinds)
Lettuce
Mushrooms (All Kinds)
Mustard Greens
Okra
Onions
Parsley
Peppers (All Kinds)
Pumpkin (not too much)
Radicchio
Radishes
Rhubarb

Romaine Lettuce
Scallion
Shallots
Seaweed (All Sea Vegetables)
Shallots
Spaghetti Squash
Spinach
Swiss Chard
Tomatoes (not too much)
Turnip Greens
Watercress
Zucchini

FERMENTED VEGETABLES
Kimchi
Sauerkraut

FRUITS

Most fruits are off limits on a ketogenic diet. Some small amounts of berries are considered ok, but watch how much you eat!

Avocado
Blackberry
Blueberry
Cranberry
Olive

Lemon
Lime
Raspberry
Strawberry

MEATS

All cuts of the animal are good to eat, but too much protein can hamper ketosis, so watch how much you eat.

Alligator	Goat	Quail
Bear	Goose	Rabbit
Beef	Horse	Sheep
Bison	Kangaroo	Snake
Chicken	Lamb	Turkey
Deer	Moose	Veal
Duck	Pheasant	Wild Boar
Elk	Pork	Wild Turkey

CURED AND PREMADE MEATS (CHECK INGREDIENTS)

All cuts of the animal are good to eat, but too much protein can hamper ketosis, so watch how much you eat.

Sausages	Pepperoni	Bacon
Deli meat	Prosciutto	
Hot dogs	Salami	

ORGAN MEATS

In the United States, organ meats have fallen out of favor, but there is no other category of food that is as nutritious. Eat any of the following from pretty much any animal.

Heart	Kidney	Tongue
Liver	Bone Marrow	Tripe

GREEN BEANS + PEAS

Almost all legumes are off limits, but small amounts of green beans and peas are ok.

FATS

Fats play a huge part in the ketogenic diet (they make up the majority of your calorie intake), so make sure you're taking in plenty of healthy fats.

Avocado Oil	Red Palm Oil	Cocoa Butter
Ghee	Palm Shortening	Walnut Oil (small amounts)
Coconut Oil	Duck Fat	Sesame Oil (small amounts)
Lard	Butter (if you tolerate dairy)	MCT Oil
Tallow	Coconut Butter	
Olive Oil		
Macadamia Oil		

the Essential KETO COOKBOOK

FISH

Fish is highly nutritious, but buy wild-caught fish whenever possible.

Anchovies
Bass
Cod
Eel
Flounder
Haddock
Halibut
Herring
Mackerel

Mahi Mahi
Mackerel
Orange Roughy
Perch
Red Snapper
Rockfish
Salmon (including Smoked Salmon)
Sardines

Tilapia
Tuna (including Albacore)
Sole
Grouper
Turbot
Trout
Shark

SHELLFISH AND OTHER SEAFOOD

Apart from organ meats, shellfish is the most nutrient-dense food you can eat. Often expensive, but worth it.

Abalone
Caviar
Clams
Crab

Lobster
Mussels
Oysters
Shrimp

Scallops
Squid

DRINKS

Watch out for hidden sugar in drinks!

Coconut Milk
Almond Milk
Cashew Milk
Broth (or bouillon)
Coffee

Tea
Herbal Teas
Water
Seltzer Water

Lemon and Lime Juice
Club Soda
Sparkling Mineral Water

NUTS AND SEEDS

Don't go wild on these as they're easy to overeat and high in omega-6 fats. These also add to your carbohydrate intake, so watch out. Lastly, note that peanut is a legume, not a nut, and is not recommended.

Almonds
Hazelnuts
Macadamias
Pecans
Pine Nuts

Pistachios
Pumpkin Seeds
Psyllium Seeds
Sesame Seeds
Sunflower Seeds

Walnuts
Cashews
Chia Seeds
Various Nut Butters

DAIRY

Not everyone can tolerate dairy - you should eliminate these foods for at least a month, then reintroduce them to see how they make you feel. We find raw and unpasteurized dairy to be better. Stick to full-fat dairy.

Kefir

Full-Fat Yogurt

Raw Full-Fat Cheeses

Full Fat Cottage Cheese

Heavy Whipping Cream

Full-Fat Sour Cream

Butter (not Margarine)

Ghee

Full-Fat Cream Cheese

HERBS AND SPICES

Experiment with these herbs and spices as they'll make your food really delicious! Make sure the check the ingredients of any herb or spice blends to avoid added sugar or MSG.

Sea Salt

Black Pepper

White Pepper

Basil

Italian Seasoning

Chili Powder

Cayenne Pepper

Curry Powder

Garam Masala

Cumin

Oregano

Thyme

Rosemary

Sage

Turmeric

Parsley

Cilantro

Cinnamon

Nutmeg

Cloves

Allspice

Ginger

Cardamom

Paprika

Dill

OTHER

These are some foods that don't fall neatly into other categories.

Pork Rinds

Beef Jerky

Pickles

Cod Liver Oil (Fish Oil)

Vinegars (check the ingredients to make sure they don't have added sugar or wheat)

Eggs (of any animal)

Salad Dressings (made with good oils and no added sugar)

Mayonnaise (made with good oils - see list of oils)

Full-fat Ranch Dressing

Caesar Dressing

Mustard

Hot Sauce (check ingredients)

Gluten Free Tamari Sauce or Coconut Aminos

Fish Sauce (check ingredients)

Cacao Nibs

Shredded Coconut

Gelatin (as a powder or from bone broth)

Vanilla Extract

Dark Chocolate (100%)

Stevia (small amounts if necessary)

Monk Fruit or Lo Han Guo Sweetener

Almond Flour or Almond Meal

Coconut Flour

Cacao Powder (unsweetened)

MORE RESOURCES

MORE RECIPES AND KETO INFO

Go to http://paleomagazine.com/ketogenic-resources and sign up for our email updates.